the energy secret

**Within each of us lies a hidden energy system:
tap into its power and you can keep yourself
healthy, happy and in perfect harmony**

the energy secret

Jane Alexander

Thorsons
Directions for Life

Thorsons
Directions for Life

Thorsons
An Imprint of HarperCollinsPublishers
77–85 Fulham Palace Road,
Hammersmith, London W6 8JB

The Thorsons website address is: www.thorsons.com

Published by Thorsons 2000
10 9 8 7 6 5 4 3 2 1

Text copyright © Jane Alexander 2000
Copyright © HarperCollinsPublishers Ltd 2000

Jane Alexander asserts the moral right to be identified as the author of this work

Editor: Nicky Vimpany
Design: XAB design
Production: Monica Green

A catalogue record for this book is available from the British Library

ISBN 0 7225 3980 0

Printed in Hong Kong

DEDICATION: For Kate and James – who personify pure energy

ACKNOWLEDGEMENTS

I have had the luck and honour to have met and learned from so many great energy workers and teachers over the years. Their wisdom infuses every page of this book and so I wholeheartedly thank them all – including (to name but a few): Denise Linn, Sarah Shurety, Keith Mason, Jane Mayers, Richard Lanham, Vera Diamond, Maurice and Nicola Griffin, Julian Baker, Gillie Gilbert, Maria Mercati, Angelika Hochadel, Jessica Loeb, Emma Field, Malcolm Kirsch, Monica Anthony, Theo Gimbel, Lynne Crawford, Sheila MacLeod, Ruth Delman and Kenneth Gibbons, Marie-Louise Lacy, Hazel Courteney, Harry Oldfield, Kenneth Meadows, Leo Rutherford, Ramses Seleem, Gina Lazenby, William Spear, Dr Rajendra Sharma, Doja Purkitt, Dr Marilyn Glenville, Jane Thurnell-Read, Christine Steward, Terry Peterson, Sue Weston, Andrew Chevalier, Michael Brookman, Karen Kingston, Liz Williams, Will Parfitt, Dee Jones, Joel Carbonnel, Simon Brown, Rosamund Webster, Paresh Rink, Ian Hayward, Margaret-Anne Pauffley and Paul Dennis, Allan Rudolf, Jennie Crewdson, Margareta Loughran, Patricia Martello, Kate Roddick, Serena Smith, Angela Renton, Susan Lever, Shan, Howard Charing, Linda Coriello and Mark Preston, Dr Tamara Voronina, Pauline Groman, Nick Williams, Ben Renshaw, Pim de Gryff, Elaine Arthey, Sebastian Pole and Jeff Lennard.

Especial thanks to Margot Gordon who planted the energy seed in my head. And to Belinda Budge of Thorsons who had the big vision and made this book happen. Also huge thanks to Nicky Vimpany, Catherine Forbes, Megan Slyfield and Hatty Madden. Bev Speight and Nigel Wright at XAB Design have made this book as beautiful as I had desired – thank you. And a big hug goes, as always, to Judy Chilcote, my agent.

Loads of love to my family and friends who provided the essential emotional energy that lies behind any book. And a heart-felt 'thank you' goes to Sarah Dening who has been a wonderful friend and great source of inspiration, support and energetic wisdom throughout the writing of this book.

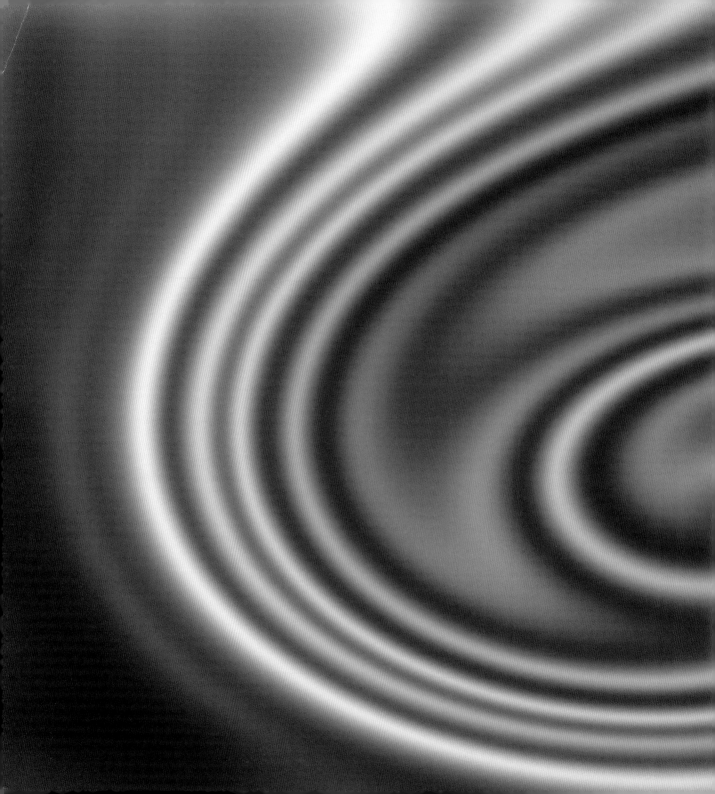

contents

WHAT IS ENERGY?

What links sex with shiatsu? What connects feng shui with cooking? Why is a business meeting similar to splashing into the sea? The answer to all these curious questions lies in one simple word: energy. Vital energy runs through all of life. It connects our bodies with our minds and souls. It links us with other people, with our homes and nature, with the universe and with the highest spiritual power.

We cannot see this subtle yet powerful force – but its effects rule every moment of our being. When our vital energy is sluggish or unawakened, life seems dull or difficult. We seem to move through life as if through treacle. Relationships seem difficult; we feel constantly under par in our bodies; work is a chore; our homes never feel quite right. On the other hand, if our energy is running out of control, life is a roller-coaster: we feel constantly stressed and strained, our nerves jangle, we seem to exist in a mêlée of arguments and irritability. However, once we start to recognize vital energy and begin to work with it, everything can change. Our lives can take on fresh meaning and purpose. When our own vital energy is moving smoothly and serenely through us, we can enjoy radiant good health, abundant vitality and a sense of ease in our bodies. Our relationships become honest, exciting and supportive. Our homes become places of serenity and joy, filled with a warm, embracing atmosphere. We start to feel a link of kinship with the whole of creation – from urban cityscape to the wild elements of nature. Work and play become intermingled – fulfilling, exciting and creative. Best of all, we no longer feel alone in a large, often frightening universe: we become linked to spirit, joined to the source of all energy.

At first the concept of energy seems rather nebulous. We talk about feeling full of energy, filled with verve, enthusiasm, pure joie de vivre. We understand the scientific concept of energy - giving power, motion, light, movement. But now we are beginning to become more aware of what is known as subtle energy or vital energy. This is the unseen force that moves throughout all of creation – through our bodies, through our houses, through the landscape, throughout the universe. This is the energy that acupuncturists speak of passing along meridians, the unseen pathways of the body. It is this energy that the clairvoyant sees as an aura, a coccoon of shimmering light around us. It is this vital energy that feng shui consultants describe as chi as it moves through our homes and environment. This is what the Indian mystics call prana, the living force that animates our food, our bodies, our relationships.

The key to getting the very best out of life lies in understanding and working with this energy. Although we cannot see it, we can most certainly feel it. Simple techniques and exercises can help you recognize the energy within your body, in those of other people, in the atmosphere of your home and the wider world. Once you can sense vital energy, you can begin to work with it – helping it move in the most beneficial way. Because energy is a natural force, left to its own devices it will, like water, take the easiest route. If nothing stands in its way it will flow smoothly and harmoniously, like a river running through a wide, straight plane. If however, it is forced into a narrow, restrictive pattern it will roar fast and furious – like a river forced between steep ravines or tumbling freefall down a mountain side. If, on the other hand, it becomes caught or entangled, it will become heavy and stagnant, like the water in a pool or a sidebend of a river, where it slowly becomes rank and murky. So our aim is to allow the vital energy around us to flow smoothly, taking away any restrictions without allowing it to run too wildly and crazily.

To choose to live with energy is to tap into an endless source of personal power and joy. It is a lifestyle choice, affecting every area of daily life in the deepest possible way. As a wonderful bodywork practitioner I know, Margot Gordon, puts it: 'We're looking at the rise of Qi Culture – acceptance and understanding of energy will infuse all our lives in every way.' I agree. In the near future, energyworking will become a familiar, accepted part of everyday life. We will think nothing of healing our bodies with energy, rather than crude medications. Ancient civilizations understood that we are not just flesh and bones; we are infused with a subtle form of energy that cannot be seen by the naked eye or under the microscope of science. Healers from China, India, Tibet and the Middle East all mapped the subtle energy centres and pathways of the body and used them for precise healing. Shamanic cultures from all around the world have shifted energy in their ceremonies, often with miraculous and seemingly inexplicable results. Some researchers and mystics even believe that long-lost civilizations, such as Atlantis, Mu and Lemuria, held the secrets of vibrational healing, turning away from surgery and drugs to use subtle energy healing methods – colour, sound, flower and gem essences.

In recent years our modern culture has begun to rediscover these long-lost methods. For many years complementary and alternative therapists have worked with subtle energy and seen with their own eyes that, by working on the esoteric level, they could bring about huge changes in the physical body. Scientists remained sceptical: no-one had ever seen a meridian, an aura, a chakra, they argued. But in recent years new, open-minded investigation into this field has shown remarkable results: you can see the aura and the subtle energy pathways. It has been proven that healers can effect physical change.

We stand on the brink of an explosion in energy medicine. In the future it will not seem strange to treat cancer with colour, rheumatism with sound. No-one will scoff at the concept of flower essences shifting emotions, homoeopathy (where not a molecule of the original substance remains) curing eczema, or acupuncture reversing infertility. Energy healers will scan our bodies for lack of balance and be able to correct it without the need for invasive surgery. Even better, we will be able to detect imbalance in ourselves and take steps to redress it – without the need to seek professional help. This will become the ultimate form of preventative medicine, gently healing emotional trauma and even genetic material before it turns pathological. We will be able to uncover and eradicate the psychospiritual traumas that underlie much of modern illness before they become a physiological problem.

The homes of the future will be havens of peace and joy. Understanding the concepts of vital energy, our architects and builders will produce homes with true spirit and soul. Decorators will realize that the colours, textures, lights and shapes they choose will affect not only our aesthetic tastes but also our moods and feelings – they will be able to tailor your home to fit your innermost needs. Simple energy techniques will enable you to create precisely the mood you need in your home – be it vibrant party place or serene sanctuary. Working with energy will allow you to guard your property and yourself as if you had an invisible safety fence.

Energy underpins relationships too. Just as we need smooth, harmonious energy flowing through our bodies and homes, we need to invest some time sensing and smoothing the energy that exists between ourselves and the people we love and work with. Whether it's your partner, child, friend or boss – when you learn how to harmonize the energy between you, your relationship will undoubtedly improve. If all of society were to learn energy healing techniques, the world would be a safer, happier, more relaxed place.

Continuing our look to the future, I would hope that an understanding of energy might bring about more respect for our environment, for the planet. When you understand how energy flows, it becomes a travesty to build houses, offices, malls in places where the Earth's energy needs to flow unrestricted. You can almost feel the Earth wince as we ride roughshod over its meandering energy pathways – clogging its 'arteries' and 'veins' with concrete and iron. A feel for its vital energy could teach us where it is right to build and where to leave nature wild and free.

At the ultimate level, cultivating energy leads to a wonderful sense of spiritual renewal. Some people have a vibrant living faith, either as part of an orthodox religion or through a private sense of belief. But many people nowadays feel alienated from traditional religions or unable to reconcile their own feelings with the dogma and rituals of age-old sects. However, once you begin to work with energy, the outward trappings of religion become unimportant. Ultimately, it doesn't matter how you perceive God, Goddess, Creator, Great Spirit – when you connect to the living, vibrant energy of the universe, there is no need for names or titles. Instead there is a wonderful sense of belonging, of love, peace and connection. As beings of energy we become united with the source of all energy and therein lies our purpose and our meaning.

The aim of this book is to introduce you to the idea of sensing, understanding and working with energy in the simplest way possible. It is inherently practical – if you want to read about the science, theory and philosophy of energy there are other books that can explain it very well. My purpose is to get you working with energy – from the very first page. Hopefully by the end of the book you will feel comfortable enough with vital energy to use its power in every area of your life. How you work with it is up to you. You may find you are interested in certain parts rather than others: you might want to look at energy in the body and not be that concerned about how it affects your home or job. That's fine – each segment stands more or less alone and you can use the information however it suits you (although I would point out that it helps to do the initial exercises before attempting any energy work). However, I suspect that, once you start working with energy in one area of your life, it will start to spill over into all parts. Energy is like that: as I've already said, it reacts like water, and have you ever tried to contain water once it spills out on a table? Before you know it, it has gone everywhere and affected everything.

Above all, I hope the process of energyworking is fun. If at any time it becomes boring or irritating or a chore, then maybe this isn't the right time for you to be attempting this work. Leave it aside and come back to it later.

Introductions over. Let's get working. Let's start feeling energy at work in our lives...

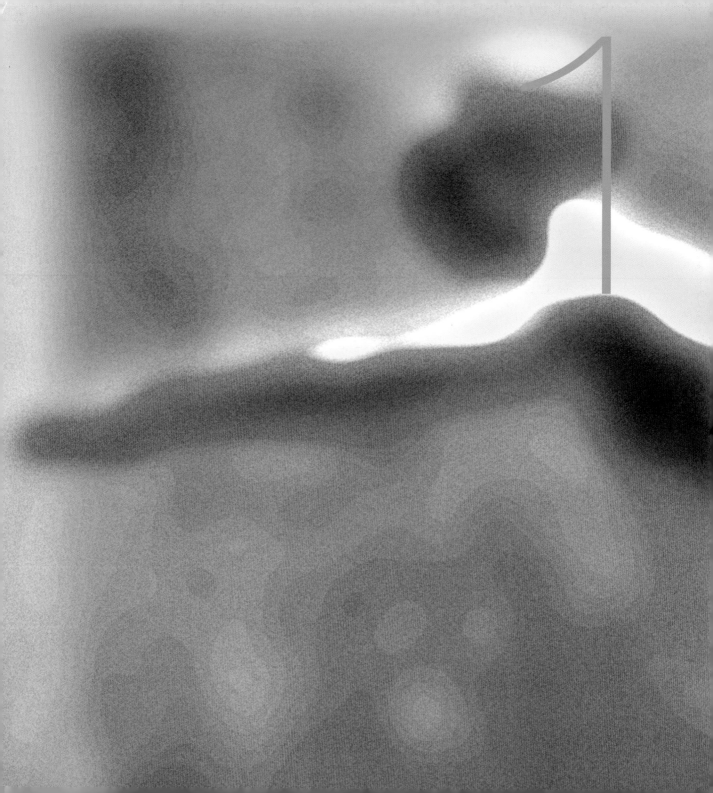

bodyenergy

CHAPTER ONE

FEELING ENERGY WITHIN THE BODY

Let's start right away by getting the smallest sense of the energy that flows all through our bodies. Take off your shoes and stand with your feet shoulder width apart. Let your knees soften and allow your hands to fall gently by your sides. Imagine you have a string coming from the top of your head, right in the centre of your scalp. It is attached to the ceiling and is gently tugging so you're totally but gently upright. Consciously relax your shoulders, your neck. Close your eyes and become aware of your breath. Just stand and breathe for a few minutes. Now become aware of the centre of your body, the area around your navel. Breathe into that area, deep strong breaths. Focus on this area being the centre of your Self. Keep breathing – slowly and steadily.

Even if you do nothing else from this book, just taking out two minutes a day to stand, centre and focus – and feel your energy – is a huge step.

How do you feel? Many people quickly start to feel a tingling through the body. This is your body's energy and it is reacting to this most simple exercise – you stopping for a moment and paying attention. Vital energy is always there – we just tend to ignore it. If you didn't feel the energy, don't panic. Not everyone does immediately. But take the odd few minutes every so often and keep trying. It will come.

Throughout the ages, people have sought to understand the complexity of the energy systems of the body. Every great culture studied the movement of energy within the body and many charted it with great precision. They believed our bodies were microcosms of the universe – that what lies without in the starry cosmos also lies within. The Qabalists, ancient Jewish mystics, taught that divine energy came down from the Godhead in a lightning flash, transforming itself from pure cosmic energy into matter. Our bodies are a miracle and a profound mystery. However much we know there is still far more that we don't. Holistic physicians are convinced that the future lies not in separating out body, mind and spirit, but understanding that they all affect each other. The burgeoning field of psychoneuroimmunology shows that what we feel and think affects our bodies. Psychologists understand that our posture can affect the way we feel and think. Bodyworkers have seen memories come flooding back when they press into muscle or connective tissue. An uplifting of the soul can have miraculous effects on disease. Prayer can heal. This is the work of energy within the body, mind and soul. Once we learn to get in touch with that energy we can start to experience our own lightning flash of pure aliveness. Let's get started...

GET IN TOUCH WITH YOUR BODY

Before we can start energy searching, we need to tackle the basics and get in touch with our bodies. Most of us don't live in our bodies; we live in our heads. We can go from one end of the day to the other without really thinking about our bodies. Sure we stop for lunch – because that's our habit. OK, we get up once in a while to go to the bathroom – our bladders are one part of our bodies it's hard to ignore. But how often do we stop and sense our bodies, think about how they feel throughout the day? Probably not much, if at all. If we want to get in touch with the vital energy of our bodies, we will need to be far more aware of what is actually going on at any one moment within our physical frames.

So stop this very moment and take an inventory. Sense how your body feels. How's your neck? Tense? Are your shoulders relaxed or up around your ears? Are you clenching your teeth so hard that your jaw is hurting? Does your body need anything? Water perhaps? Food? (Often our bodies are just plain hungry or hungry for food that really sustains. Some fruit or a proper lunch of soup, wholemeal bread and salad rather than a limp sandwich.) Have you been sitting so long that your back aches or your buttocks are numb? Do you need a good stretch? Do your eyes feel bright or sore and itchy? If you stare at a computer screen all day, do your eyes need to rest or to focus on something long distance? Are you tired? Does your whole body need a quick catnap or a longer rest?

Of course it won't always be possible to give your body precisely what it needs, but try to give it something, even if it is just a quick fix. If you work on a computer you can programme your machine to beep at given intervals. You could set it up for once every thirty minutes or, at the least, every hour. Then quickly run through your body and see what it needs. At the very minimum give yourself a drink of mineral water and a quick stretch. Get up, walk around a bit or do some simple neck rolls. You'll find your work easier if your body is relaxed and happy. You don't need a computer for this: set your watch or alarm clock – or even the oven timer – to give you hourly warnings. If you're a busy mother or work manually your body will be asking for different things – probably rest, a couple of minutes' sit-down. But stretching and water will probably make your body smile whatever you do.

Also, try to set aside a small amount of time every day to re-establish true, meaningful contact with your body. These exercises can help.

exercise

PAYING ATTENTION EXERCISE
Wearing loose clothes and no shoes, lie on the floor on your back. Become aware of your body lying on the floor – feel the floor under you and where it supports your body. Now put your attention in your feet – imagine the bones of your feet, the muscles, the tendons, the skin. Are they hot or cold? Do you feel any difference between your two feet? Are they light or heavy? Now gradually work your way up the body, repeating the questions, becoming aware of how different parts of your body feel. Move up your legs and into the hips, up the torso and into the abdomen, the chest and the shoulders. Then down the arms into the hands. Finish by examining your head and face.

BONE-BALANCING
Now get the energy moving through your skeleton, your bone structure. Use either your lightly clenched fists or your fingers and swiftly tap over your hip-bones and pelvis. Listen to the sound it makes and feel the vibration in your body. Move down your legs and listen and feel for changes in sound and feeling. Try the soles of your feet. Work over all the bones in your body, noting differences.

HEART SEARCHING
Just take a moment to think about your heart. Sit quietly and start to listen for its beat. Tune in to its rhythm. If you feel comfortable with this (not everyone will) let yourself focus further on the heart – go inside it, feel it pulsing. Listen to the blood sluicing through its valves, pumping life and energy out and towards every cell in your body. How do you feel? What are your thoughts?

The first time I tried this exercise I experienced an incredible connection with my heart. For the first time in my life I was aware of (and quite bowled over by) its stoic power; its faithful toil. I felt humbled and grateful. Then I felt that I never wanted to hurt my heart again: I wanted to help it, rather than hinder it. I wanted to give it the food and exercise it needs to function with ease. It was a turning point for me.

If you are one of the many people who feel uncomfortable or even nauseous at the thought of 'going inside' your heart, don't worry. It's quite a common feeling. Sometimes it can evoke feelings of panic or distaste. For the moment, don't worry about it – just let it go. You might try the exercise later on and find a quite different reaction.

exercise

FIND YOUR OTHER ORGANS

If you felt comfortable with the heart exercise, you can follow the same technique for getting in touch with other organs. Follow your breathing to bring yourself into your lungs. Feel them expand and contract, pulling air into the tiny sacs. Imagine the exchange of gases and then the oxygenated blood flowing out to all the cells. Remember that your lungs connect you with the outside world. They are also literally inspirers – you pull in love of life, energy, enthusiasm; you breathe out the old, the expired, waste. Feel how your body breathes for you; it actually breathes you. You can continue this exercise to other parts of your body, other organs. What do you discover?

If you don't feel comfortable exploring your body in this way, gently ask yourself why this is. Does it bring back any uncomfortable memories? Is it frightening? See if you can work out why this should be. You might want just to try this exercise every day – see if the feelings change. If, on the other hand, you're just not ready for this, don't worry about it. When the time is right, you'll be able to go into your body feeling fine and comfortable.

Our bodies are not just composed of flesh and blood, they are complex chemical factories and, above all, energy powerhouses, sources of spirit

BREATHING – A DIRECT ROUTE TO ENERGYWORKING

Once you have started a relationship with your body, you are ready to move one step further on the energy route. Breathing techniques are some of the oldest and most effective ways of awakening, stimulating, balancing and soothing energy within the body and mind. Breathing is powerful medicine. The Eastern arts of yoga and chi kung have developed a whole science of breathing and promise that particular forms of breathing can do everything from improving your mood to increasing your resistance to colds and illness and even helping you resist ageing. Good breathing feeds the brain, calms the nerves and has a measurable effect on a number of medical conditions.

Once you start breathing properly, you should notice changes – often profound changes. Symbolically, breathing is all about taking in the new and eliminating the old. The Buddhist tradition regards every breath as giving new life and every exhalation as a little death. So, taking in deep joyful breaths is seen as a way of affirming life and vitality. There is a yoga proverb that says: 'Life is in the breath. Therefore he who only half breathes, half lives.' Let's look at some simple breathing exercises, which will help you become more adept at recognizing and shifting energy within the body.

THE COMPLETE BREATH

This is the basic breathing technique of pranayama, the yogic science of breathing. It is an excellent training tool as it encourages you to breathe fully, bringing oxygen deep into the cells and pulling out toxins. It will also send a surge of energy through every cell of your body.

1. Lie down on the floor and make yourself comfortable. Bring your feet close in to your buttocks, with the soles of the feet together, and allow the knees to fall apart, hands resting gently on your abdomen. (Note: if this feels uncomfortable you can put cushions under your knees.) This posture stretches the lower abdomen, which enhances the breathing process.

2. Breathe in with a slow, smooth inhalation through your nostrils, feeling your abdomen expand and contract. Your fingers will part as your abdomen expands.

3. Exhale slowly and steadily through your nostrils. Notice that your abdomen flattens and your fingers are touching.

exercise

4. Pause for a second or two and then repeat this inhalation and exhalation, becoming conscious of the movement of the breath down through your chest and abdomen. Breathe naturally at your own pace in this way for five minutes or as long as you feel comfortable.

5. If you feel comfortable with this you can extend the breath so it comes up from the abdomen into the chest as you inhale. This provides a longer, deeper breath.

6. Finally, bring your knees together and gently stretch out the legs. Allow yourself to relax comfortably on the ground for a few minutes (you may feel more comfortable with a cushion under your lower back or your neck).

ALTERNATE NOSTRIL BREATHING
This exercise stimulates the two hemispheres of the brain and helps bring them into balance. Therefore it is very harmonizing and soothing to both the brain and the body. It brings a wonderful sense of calm, focused energy – I would recommend trying this exercise whenever you need to soothe yourself, whether physically or emotionally, or if you cannot sleep ...

1. Sit comfortably in a chair, with both feet on the floor. Don't slouch. Gently allow your eyes to close, your body to relax and your mind to still.

2. Place your dominant hand around your nose. If you are right-handed the most natural way to do this will be to rest your right thumb against your right nostril with the rest of the fingers lying gently towards your left nostril. The aim is to close off one nostril at a time, comfortably and easily, without constantly moving your hand.

3. Close the right nostril gently and slowly exhale through your left nostril. Note that you are starting the breath on an exhale. Then inhale through the same nostril.

4. Swap nostrils by exhaling through the right and inhaling again. Don't try to breathe very deeply – keep it natural. You may find you need to blow your nose a lot – don't worry, that's perfectly normal.

5. Alternate between the two nostrils for around five minutes if you can. If you feel uncomfortable at any time, breathe through your mouth for a while until you can go back to the nose.

6. When you've finished, allow yourself to simply relax with your eyes closed for a while.

exercise

exercise

THE DETOX BREATH

This powerful breathing sends your energy into battle against toxins. It is said to strengthen the lungs, to massage and tone the abdominal muscles and refresh the nervous system. However it IS strong medicine and should not be used if you have a heart condition, high blood pressure, epilepsy, hernia or any ear, nose or eye problems; if you are pregnant or menstruating.

1. Choose your position. This exercise can be performed sitting, standing or lying down. Make sure you are comfortable and relaxed. Breathe regularly and normally.

2. Inhale slowly, smoothly and deeply, but do not strain your breathing.

3. Now exhale briskly, as if you were sneezing. Focus your attention on your abdomen – it will automatically flatten and tighten as you exhale.

4. Allow yourself to inhale naturally – it will happen automatically following the brisk exhale.

5. Now continue breathing in this way for a few minutes – or as you feel comfortable. It is a brisk, energetic technique so don't be surprised if you only manage a minute or so to begin with.

6. Resume normal breathing and relax.

> **NOTE:** If you are pregnant or menstruating you can use a modified form of this exercise. Instead of the 'sneezing' exhale, pout your lips and allow your breath to come out in a steady stream, as if you were blowing out candles on a cake. This is a much slower technique than the basic detox breath but still excellent.

UJJAYI – THE VICTORIOUS BREATH

Use this yogic breathing technique whenever you need to calm down. It sends a soothing stream of energy throughout the body and mind. It is an important technique that we will need to use when we discuss using exercise to raise energy – so take some time to get to grips with it.

1. Learn how to practise ujjayi sitting comfortably with your eyes gently shut. With a little practice you can use ujjayi in any position.

2. Breathe in deeply, contracting the muscles around the top of your windpipe. Focus on your throat and you should hear a gentle hissing sound.

exercise

3. Now breathe out as slowly as possible, closing off the muscles around the epiglottis. Your breath will sound rasping, as if you had a bad cold.

4. Breathe in and out in this way six times.

5. Now relax and breathe normally.

6. If you have time, repeat this cycle (six ujjayi breaths then six normal breaths) for four cycles.

THE YOGIC COOLING BREATH

This breath is also very soothing and relaxing – ideal for when you feel overheated and irritable. It is also a very simple way to feel energy moving down the spine and throughout the whole body.

1. Sit down in a comfortable position. Place your hands softly on your knees. Close your eyes and become aware of your natural breathing pattern.

2. Curl up your tongue into a tube, letting the tip protrude slightly out of your lips. If you cannot do this just keep your mouth slightly open and allow the air to come in over your tongue.

3. Breathe in slowly and deeply through the gap in your tongue. You will feel a cool rush of air on your tongue.

4. Now breathe out in the same way, slowly and deeply. Continue like this for a few minutes, or as long as you feel comfortable. You should notice a cooling effect down the spine and spreading out through the entire body.

5. Return to normal breathing, focusing on your natural breath. Once again, become aware of your surroundings.

6. Cast your gaze down and slowly open your eyes. Focus on how you feel: sit still for a few moments and feel how the energy in your body has shifted.

CAUTION
These breathing exercises can be a very powerful process. Anyone with any chest problems should take the exercises very slowly and carefully, preferably under the guidance of a trained yoga or chi kung teacher. Anyone with a heart condition, blood pressure problems or glaucoma should not hold the breath – again consult a trained teacher. If in any doubt, consult your physician or a trained practitioner.

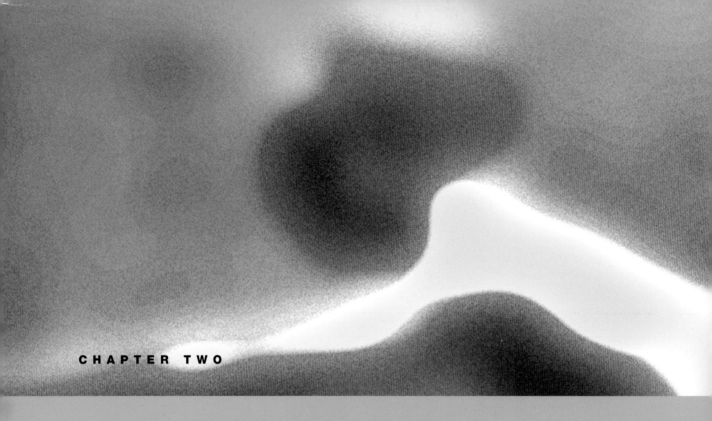

CHAPTER TWO

AURAS AND CHAKRAS

In the last chapter we looked at some very simple but effective ways of getting in touch with the energy within our bodies. If you take the time to practise them regularly you will come to feel the unmistakable surge of vital energy as it courses through your body. With more practice you will be able to direct this energy to particular parts of your body. We will look at this further on in this chapter as we investigate the energy centres of the body, the chakras.

Simply by breathing, you will be able to bring a sparkle of energy tingling through you, as if you were standing under an exhilarating mountain waterfall.

But to begin with, we're going to look at the aura, the area of subtle energy that vibrates around our bodies. It is what we recognize as a halo around the heads of very spiritual beings such as Christ, Buddha, Mohammed and Vishnu. But you don't have to be a highly evolved spiritual leader to have an aura. Each and every one of us has this energy, it's just that few know how to see it. Once you learn to see the aura (and it's quite a simple process) you have a unique insight into yourself and the people around you. Reading auras could warn you away from unscrupulous people. It could also let you know when someone is angry, jealous or lying. By catching the clues in the aura, you could stop rows before they even start. You would know when to give your partner kind, loving support when he or she were feeling low.

The aura cannot lie. The almost 'chemical' reaction we often experience (love at first sight, loathing at first sight!) could be due to how our aura reacts to someone else's. If someone feels uncomfortable, their aura will 'shrink' away from the other person's. If one person is pushy and aggressive, their aura can envelop the other's. On the other hand, people who feel comfortable together will show auras that happily meet or even merge into one.

Learning how to read auras is great fun – but it's not just a party trick. When you can read an aura, you can gain a huge amount of knowledge about someone – their mood, their feelings, their innermost thoughts. This can certainly help you know how best to deal with them – as we'll see in Part Two – Emotional Energy. But on a more fundamental level, learning how to sense auras is another step on the path to becoming at home with the subtle energy of the body.

HOW TO START SEEING AURAS

Virtually everyone can learn to see an aura. When I first started I trained myself by looking first at the auras of trees – they tend to be very clear. Simply pick a healthy tree at some distance from you and gaze softly at it, slightly unfocusing your eyes. You should start to see a faint shimmering of energy around the tree – that's its aura. From here, you can practise on plants. Look at the aura of a healthy plant and compare it with that of a wilted or dying plant. Next move on to animals – see if you can detect any differences between your pets. Animals are very sensitive – you can give a cat an 'aura stroke' by 'stroking' about an inch or so above its fur – often the cat will start to purr as if you were physically touching it.

SEEING SOMEONE ELSE'S AURA

When you feel confident with seeing auras on plants and animals, you can progress to reading the auras of people. If you have a willing guinea pig you can practise in a formal manner. Ask them to stand about two feet in front of a bare white wall. Position yourself a fair distance away from your guinea pig – ten feet is ideal. Look past the person's head and shoulders and focus on the wall behind, slightly unfocusing your eyes. You should start to see a thin band of fuzzy light around the person. Continue to look past the outline of the body and you might start to see shimmering colours. This is harder and can take some time to perfect. But the great thing about reading auras is that you can practise anytime – on the train, waiting in line, sitting in a restaurant, waiting for a friend. After a while you should start to notice differences between auras – some might seem brighter, others more dingy or muddy. You might notice particular colours or flashes of colour.

SEEING YOUR OWN AURA

You can also train yourself to check out your own aura. Stand in front of a mirror, as far away as possible. Again, try to have a white wall about two feet behind you – you could always hang up a sheet. Breathe calmly and focus on the wall, rather than yourself, softly defocusing your eyes. Look for colours in the aura. If you can't 'see' any colours, do you get any feelings about what colours might be there?

WHAT THE COLOURS IN AN AURA MEAN

Once you become adept at seeing auras, you will notice that they display various colours – sometimes bright and clear, sometimes muddy or cloudy. Generally speaking, a colourful, clean and bright aura shows someone who is happy and healthy. Dirty, dark colours tend to suggest either physical illness, tiredness or some kind of emotional black cloud. Experts say that the odd flash of colour in an aura could indicate an emotion that is not under control.

PURPLE/VIOLET: mysticism and spirituality. Shows a person who might be very religious, idealistic and spiritual.

INDIGO: inspiration, wisdom, sensitivity and self-mastery. Like violet, indigo also shows spiritual concerns and a devotional nature.

BLUE: strong intellect, intelligence, rational and logical thinking. Clear blue indicates intuition. Darker shades can indicate suspicion. Steely blue-grey indicates caution and control.

TURQUOISE: a dynamic person with hoards of energy. A good organizer, someone who likes to influence others. Communicative.

GREEN: green is a restful, healing colour, which shows a strong sense of balance and a deep inner calm. Kind, caring and gentle. Dark green shades in the aura, or the occasional dark green flash across the aura can warn of deceit or jealousy.

YELLOW: fun, happy, loving, cheerful personalities full of joy, freedom and vitality, compassion and optimism. Dark dull yellow points to suspicion while a dirty yellow can indicate pain or a hidden source of anger.

ORANGE: shows someone who is full of vitality, warmth and generosity. Someone who has power and who can be full of inspiration. Too much orange in the aura can indicate pride.

GOLD: A little gold in the aura is a good sign – gold usually indicates someone who is well-balanced, kind and generous. However a totally gold aura is usually only found in great spiritual leaders.

RED: Red signifies physical life, vitality, ambition and sexual power. People with lots of red in their auras are often very sensual and have a high sex drive. Dark or cloudy red can point to violent tendencies or hidden anger.

PINK: Pink is the colour of true romantic love. It also indicates modesty, shyness and gentleness.

BROWN: Not a good sign in the aura, dirty, dull brown shows an unsettled, materialistic tendency. This could be someone who is generally negative or just happens to be in a bad mood at the time!

GREY: Grey can indicate depression, fear, morbid thoughts and low energy levels.

BLACK: a pure black aura is a clear warning sign – this person has deep problems or could be a very unpleasant character. Dull murky black can indicate depression, anxiety and fear. It may also indicate illness or someone who takes drugs.

WHITE: Curiously white can have similar correspondences to black – possible illness or drug abuse.

OPAQUE COLOURS: If the colours in the aura are opaque or misty, this tends to show unresolved situations or struggle.

CLEAR, TRANSPARENT COLOURS: Clear bright colours are a good sign. Generally speaking they show someone with nothing to hide and a sunny, happy disposition.

Remember these are only guidelines – not a prescription. So use them as a starting point and then gently question your 'subject' to find out if your aura-reading is on target. Also, if you do find you have a gift for this work and can be very accurate, use your talent wisely and respectfully. Nobody likes to feel they are an open book – so I don't recommend you rush in and recommend someone has counselling for their 'drug problem' or that you warn them about the perils of being too materialistic!

BALANCE YOUR CHAKRAS FOR HEALTH AND HARMONY

Eastern religions teach that the human body contains numerous spinning spheres of bio-energetic energy, known as chakras. The seven most important ones run in a direct line from the base of the spine to the crown of the head. While scientists insist chakras don't exist because they cannot be seen under the microscope, clairvoyants claim they can easily 'see' the chakras. And the PIP scanner, which takes information from sound and light frequencies in the body, now shows what the mystics have known all along: oscillating spheres of energy in a vertical line down the body.

It's a little like tuning into a radio station: if you're on the wrong frequency the sound is distorted and unpleasant; once you hit the right frequency it becomes as clear as a bell.

The chakras are precise monitors of our physical and mental well-being. Each is said to spin at a different frequency and when each chakra spins at its perfect frequency the systems of the body radiate perfect health; emotions are centered and balanced and we enjoy optimum health and a deep sense of peace. It's a little like tuning into a radio station: if you're on the wrong frequency the sound is distorted and unpleasant; once you hit the right frequency it becomes as clear as a bell. However, with all the stresses and strains of modern life it is easy for the chakras to fall out of frequency. When this happens we either fall prey to illnesses, feel under par, or we lose our emotional equilibrium.

Learning to 'read' your chakras is actually very simple. Each chakra governs specific parts of the body and specific emotions: there are clear signs to tell whether that chakra is balanced or whether you have too much or too little energy there. Once you have worked out which chakras are unbalanced, you can redress the balance and bring them back into harmony

Within each of us lies a hidden energy system:
tap into its power and you can keep yourself healthy

happy and in perfect harmony

exercise

GETTING IN TOUCH WITH CHAKRA ENERGY

This simple exercise helps you become aware of the energy moving through the chakras. It allows you to forge strong links with Heaven above and the Earth below. It also stimulates a kind of free dialogue between the chakras. Many of us tend to be 'split' – we either live with our heads in the clouds or we are rooted to the Earth, with our feet so solidly in the mud that we cannot raise our eyes to the stars. In an ideal world we have balance – we stand firmly on the Earth but take our inspiration from Heaven.

1. Stand comfortably with your feet shoulder-width apart. As we did at the beginning of Chapter One, imagine you have a string coming from the top of your head, gently pulling you upwards. Let your knees relax, your pelvis relax, your shoulders relax. Check your jaw and make sure you aren't holding any tension there.

2. Gently close your eyes and become aware of your breathing. Don't try to force it, just be aware. You may well find it automatically starts to slow down as you relax.

3. Now imagine that above your head there is a shining ball of pure energy. If it helps you can see it as a shimmering violet colour. Imagine you are breathing into that ball. Continue this for a few breaths.

4. Now breathe in, taking in the brilliant shimmering energy from this sphere. As you breathe out, imagine the energy moving smoothly down through your body, leaving through your feet into the earth. Repeat five times.

5. Next, visualize another ball of energy, this time radiating up from the Earth to the base of your spine. This energy sphere pulsates with a steady beat, like a slow heartbeat. If you like you can imagine it as a deep, beautiful red. Breathe into this sphere slowly and steadily. You may find your breathing slows even further.

6. Now as you breathe in, take the steady red energy up through your body, up to the very top of your head. Repeat this five times.

7. Stand still for a few moments and allow your breathing to return to its usual pace. You may feel energy tingling or pulsing in your body – notice where and how it feels.

LOOKING AT THE CHAKRAS

You have just experienced, in a very small way, the energy of the chakras – in particular the crown chakra (at the top of the head) and the base chakra (at the base of the spine). Now let's take a little time to become acquainted with all seven of the major energy centres of the body. I've outlined some general guidelines, which can give an indication of whether you have an excess or deficiency of energy in any of your chakras – also some practical ways of balancing each chakra.

The Base Chakra

The base chakra is located at the base of the spine; the colour associated with it is red. This chakra governs the material world, our physical structure and our social position in life.

WHEN ITS ENERGY IS BALANCED: A well balanced base chakra brings good health and high levels of energy. You have a sense of ease and relaxation in your body and feel safe and protected in the world. You should have a secure position in the world and be materially comfortable, with enough money and possessions to enjoy a contented life.

WHEN ITS ENERGY IS DEFICIENT: You may feel disconnected from your body, you may possibly be underweight. You have a lack of focus and discipline and are very disorganized. You're fearful, anxious, restless – you can't settle. You may have money worries.

WHEN ITS ENERGY IS EXCESSIVE: You may well be overweight through overeating. You have a tendency to hoard and be greedy. Energy levels are low and you often feel sluggish and lazy. You are scared of change and crave security.

PHYSICAL EFFECTS OF IMBALANCE: Disorders of the bowel and intestines; problems with bones and teeth; eating disorders; problems with legs, feet, knees, base of spine and buttocks.

HOW TO HEAL THE BASE CHAKRA: You need to reconnect with your body. Start by doing as much physical exercise as possible – choose a sport or activity you enjoy. Try massage – find a professional aromatherapist or bodyworker or ask a friend or partner to give you massage. Yoga would be excellent as it heals and balances all the chakras. Gardening and pottery are good grounding exercises if the energy of your base chakra is deficient. On a psychological level, look at your early relationship with your mother: talk to her about it if you can – if it's painful, talk to a trained therapist or counsellor.

The Sacral Chakra

The second chakra is located between the lower abdomen and the navel. Its colour is orange. It deals with issues of sensuality and sexuality, of partnership and relationships.

WHEN ITS ENERGY IS BALANCED: A well balanced sacral chakra gives grace to your movements. You are kind to yourself and to others. Your emotions are balanced and you can enjoy pleasure without guilt.

WHEN ITS ENERGY IS DEFICIENT: Too little energy in this chakra may cause rigidity in the body and mind. There can be a fear of change and a denial of pleasure – also poor social skills. You have a general lack of desire, passion and excitement in life. You may lack interest in sex.

WHEN ITS ENERGY IS EXCESSIVE: You may well be addicted to pleasure and sex. You might be ruled by excessive emotions, swinging wildly between moods, having endless crises. Emotionally you are over-sensitive and over-dependent on others.

PHYSICAL EFFECTS OF IMBALANCE: Disorders of the reproductive and urinary systems; menstrual problems; lack of flexibility in the lower back and knees; sexual dysfunction; loss of appetite.

HOW TO HEAL THE SACRAL CHAKRA: Learn to trust and enjoy your senses – feel the textures around you; listen to new music and sounds; look at nature and at art; taste different foods and drinks. Dance can help to liberate this chakra – so can bodywork. Gently try to get in touch with your emotions (with professional help if necessary) to release any old feelings of hurt, anger and guilt.

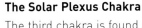

The Solar Plexus Chakra

The third chakra is found around the solar plexus area. Its colour is yellow. This chakra deals with issues of self-esteem, energy, will, confidence and inner power.

WHEN ITS ENERGY IS BALANCED: A well balanced solar plexus chakra makes for a very sunny disposition. You have plenty of self-esteem and a sense of warmth and confidence; a good sense of humour and the ability to be spontaneous and playful. You can meet challenges and are responsible and reliable. You have a sense of your own worth and power but can be disciplined when necessary.

WHEN ITS ENERGY IS DEFICIENT: Too little energy in this chakra can result in lack of physical and emotional energy, poor self-discipline and low self-esteem. You could be unreliable and overly passive, easily manipulated and a 'victim', always blaming others.

WHEN ITS ENERGY IS EXCESSIVE: You may well be aggressive and domineering, manipulative, deceitful and controlling. You have to have the last word and are prone to temper tantrums and outbursts. You have driving ambition, are very competitive and arrogant, and exceedingly stubborn.

PHYSICAL EFFECTS OF IMBALANCE: Digestive disorders and eating disorders, ulcers, muscular problems, chronic fatigue, hypertension, problems with the stomach, pancreas, gall bladder and liver, diabetes and hypoglycemia. Disorders of the reproductive and urinary systems; menstrual problems; lack of flexibility in the lower back and knees; sexual dysfunction; loss of appetite.

HOW TO HEAL THE SOLAR PLEXUS CHAKRA: If you have a deficiency you must learn how to take risks. You need grounding and emotional warmth. If you have excess of this chakra look at stress management techniques (meditation, autogenic training, etc) and deep relaxation. Anyone with problems in this chakra would benefit from doing sit-ups (abdominal crunches) to strengthen that area. Martial arts such as Judo or Tai Chi would be excellent. Psychotherapy can help you build up the necessary strength to release or contain anger and strengthen your sense of autonomy.

The Heart Chakra

The fourth chakra is based in the heart and chest. Its colour is green and it deals with issues of love, intimacy, balance and relationships.

WHEN ITS ENERGY IS BALANCED: A well balanced heart chakra makes you compassionate and loving, empathetic and altruistic, peaceful and balanced.

WHEN ITS ENERGY IS DEFICIENT: Too little energy in this chakra can make you antisocial and withdrawn, critical and judgmental of others or yourself. It can cause depression, loneliness and a fear of relationships.

WHEN ITS ENERGY IS EXCESSIVE: You may well be demanding and clinging, jealous and dependent; overly self-sacrificing.

PHYSICAL EFFECTS OF IMBALANCE: Disorders of the heart, lungs, breasts and arms. Shortness of breath and asthma. Circulation problems, immune system deficiency and tension between the shoulder blades. Pains in the chest.

HOW TO HEAL THE HEART CHAKRA: Breathing exercises will help all those with problems in the heart chakra – join a yoga or chi kung class that teaches breathing. Start a journal – writing down all your feelings and thoughts honestly. Look at your relationships and try to free yourself from suppressed grief and loss. Start to accept yourself – just as you are

The Throat Chakra

The fifth chakra is located in the throat. Its colour is blue and it deals with issues of communication and creativity.

WHEN ITS ENERGY IS BALANCED: A well balanced throat chakra shows in a resonant voice and clear communication. You should have a great sense of timing and rhythm, be a good listener and have plenty of creativity in your life.

WHEN ITS ENERGY IS DEFICIENT: If you have difficulty putting your feelings into words, or are scared of speaking out, you may be deficient in this chakra. You could be introverted and shy. Anyone who feels they are tone deaf or lacking rhythm should look at this chakra.

WHEN ITS ENERGY IS EXCESSIVE: You talk too much and can't listen. You gossip and interrupt and are known for your loud, intrusive voice.

PHYSICAL EFFECTS OF IMBALANCE: Disorders of the throat, ears, voice and neck. Tightness of the jaw.

HOW TO HEAL THE THROAT CHAKRA: If your throat chakra is deficient, you need to use your voice: singing, chanting, humming or shouting. Sound therapy or voicework would be wonderful. If you have excessive energy here, practise the art of silence and concentrate on what others are saying. All problems in this chakra would benefit from bodywork or massage.

The Brow Chakra

The sixth chakra is based in the forehead. Its colour is indigo and it deals with imagination, intuition, dreams and insights.

WHEN ITS ENERGY IS BALANCED: A well balanced brow chakra makes you intuitive and perceptive, with a good imagination. You find it simple to visualize.

WHEN ITS ENERGY IS DEFICIENT: Poor memory, vision and lack of imagination indicate a deficient brow chakra. You find it hard to remember dreams and can't envisage the future. You may be rigid in your thoughts, thinking there is only one way to do something.

WHEN ITS ENERGY IS EXCESSIVE: You live too much in your imagination – you have difficulty concentrating and have frequent nightmares. You may be obsessive and even suffer delusions.

PHYSICAL EFFECTS OF IMBALANCE: Headaches, poor eyesight or problems with vision.

HOW TO HEAL THE BROW CHAKRA: Try painting and drawing – use whatever materials and colours you like and paint whatever comes to mind. Start to write down and work with your dreams. Try meditation or autogenic training.

The Crown Chakra

The seventh chakra is found in the cerebral cortex in the brain. Its colour is violet and it rules understanding and our connection with God and the divine.

WHEN ITS ENERGY IS BALANCED: A well balanced crown chakra will allow you to be open-minded, intelligent, thoughtful and wise. You can analyze and assimilate information easily. You have broad understanding and will generally have a sense of spiritual connection.

WHEN ITS ENERGY IS DEFICIENT: You are cynical and tend to ridicule spirituality. Your belief systems are very rigid. You may be apathetic. You could be greedy and materialistic.

WHEN ITS ENERGY IS EXCESSIVE: You are too intellectual and live in your head. You have lost touch with your body and may be excessively spiritual and confused.

PHYSICAL EFFECTS OF IMBALANCE: Migraines, amnesia.

HOW TO HEAL THE CROWN CHAKRA: Meditation could be very useful. Be open to new ideas and new information. Examine your attitudes to spirituality and religion. If you have an excess of crown chakra energy you need to connect with your body and the Earth – try physical exercise, massage or gardening. If you have a deficiency, open yourself to the idea of spirituality, allow yourself to drop your cynicism and have an open mind.

exercise

CONTACTING THE CHAKRAS THROUGH SOUND

Each chakra has its own sound. By toning the sounds of the chakras we can get in touch with the chakras and feel their individual energies.

1. Stand or sit comfortably. Take a few deep groans to release your jaw and neck. Yawn to loosen your mouth. When you feel ready, close your eyes and focus on your breathing. As you become aware of your breath, take it down to your abdomen, so you are breathing fully.

2. Start by visualizing your base chakra pulsing steadily, deep red in the base of your spine. Breathe into the chakra and, when you feel ready, start to tone the sound 'uh' (like a deep groan). Make it as deep and resonant as you can. Imagine the sound coming from your base chakra. As one 'uh' ends, breathe and start another. Keep going for as long as feels comfortable – around two minutes is ideal.

3. Now visualize your sacral chakra, glowing orange, about three inches below the navel. Breathe into this chakra and tone its sound which is 'oooo' – still a deep sound but not as profound as the 'uh'. Can you feel this sound resonate in your genital area?

4. The next chakra is the solar plexus chakra – between your ribs and naval. It is a pure bright yellow and its sound is a mid-range 'oh' (rhyming with so and go).

5. Bring your awareness up into your heart chakra, which shines with a soft green. The sound is a soft and gentle 'ah' (as in father). Is the sound resonating in your heart? If not, imagine it is.

6. Move to your throat chakra, which glimmers pure blue. The sound is 'eye' as in the word 'I'. It is higher in tone, clear and almost perlucid. Hear the sound vibrating through your body.

7. The sixth chakra is located at the site of the third eye – in the centre of your forehead. It shines with a pure indigo. Tone the sound 'ey' (as in say). Feel your third eye energized by the sound, your intuition enlivened.

8. The last chakra is the crown chakra and is located at the top of your head. It shimmers with a beautiful purple light. The sound here is the highest of all – a gentle, not shrill, 'eee' (as in me, he, be). Feel that sound resonating in your crown chakra.

9. Now imagine your toning linking all the chakras together, so there is a glistening bolt of energy running right through the centre of your body.

10. Stand or sit quietly when you have finished and slowly allow yourself to come back to waking consciousness. Stamp your feet to ground yourself – you may need something to eat too.

MOVING ENERGY WITHIN THE BODY

Now we are able to start consciously directing energy within the body.

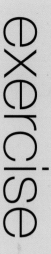

1. Stand comfortably with your feet shoulder-width apart and relax as for the previous exercise. Close your eyes and become aware of your breathing. You may find it automatically starts to slow down as you become relaxed and quiet.

2. Now one-by-one we're going to contact the chakras. Start from the top and work down.

3. Start with the crown chakra. Imagine it spinning just above your head. Breathe into its pure vibrant energy. Remember it is violet and, if you like, you can also include its sound. Stay with this chakra for a few minutes, gaining a sense of how it feels.

4. Breathe in, taking in the brilliant energy from this sphere. As you breathe out, imagine the energy moving down and joining that of the next chakra, at the third eye (between your eyebrows). Breathe into this chakra, remembering it is indigo. Tone its sound, if you like.

5. Again, breathe in and move to the next chakra, at the throat. How does this chakra feel? Be aware of any nuances, any intuitions you may feel at each stage.

6. Next take the breath to your heart. Does your heart feel open? Too open maybe? Or do you feel you close it off to avoid possible hurt?

7. Now we move to the solar plexus chakra. What can you feel here – in the very centre of your being? Spend some time with each chakra – don't race through this exercise.

8. Shift the energy to the sacral chakra. What feelings do you have? Any impressions?

9. Finally, take the energy right down to the base chakra. What do you detect here?

10. Now, if you can, imagine all the chakras spinning in your body. If it's too hard to visualize all their different colours, simplify them and imagine them all as glowing white.

11. To finish, stand still for a few moments and allow your breathing to return to its usual pace. Open your eyes and stamp your feet. Have a glass of water and something to eat.

You will find that, as you become familiar with this exercise, you will be able to detect if any of your chakras are out of balance. You might see one spinning at an unusual speed, slower or faster than usual. It might seem to spin in a lopsided fashion, like a top winding down. This will give you an indication of which chakras need attention.

CHAPTER THREE

HEALING THERAPIES FOR THE BODY

We certainly have physical bodies – we can feel them and touch them. But, as I hope by now you're realizing, we are far more than mere skin and bones. We are not just a fermenting pool of biochemicals, we are, above all, energy beings. You have felt energy moving within your body. You may even have been able to move the energy in your body from one chakra to another or to bring the energy in one chakra back to balance. Energy medicine does precisely what you have been doing already with this book – it seeks to find the imbalances within your energy fields, pathways and centres and to bring them back to balance. The ways it uses to do this vary considerably but the aim is always the same – a harmonious, healthful flow of vital energy.

For millennia ancient healing systems have known about vital energy. The Chinese call it chi or qi, the Japanese ki, the Indians know it as prana, in the Middle East it is known as quwa. They mapped it clearly: the Chinese saw the body as a shimmering mass of organized energy, flowing along subtle lines – the meridians. They used pressure and fine needles to stimulate or regulate the energy at precise points along these meridians. The Indian system talks of the chakras and the nadi, channels of subtle energy or prana.

More modern systems, such as Zero Balancing and Polarity Therapy, also see energy as a complex web, existing in a vast complexity of forms and on many distinct levels. Unfortunately modern medicine hasn't adequately charted this energetic system – yet. And most modern physicians won't treat what they can't see under a microscope. Yet we ignore our energy bodies at a very high cost. Our subtle energy is our life-force, it is the very stuff that animates us. It has only been very recently that modern scientists have come to accept that mind can influence body; that spiritual well-being can have an effect on our physiological health. Mind is simply one aspect of energy; soul or spirit is another.

Imbalance always occurs first in the energetic body – stress, unhealthy thought patterns, negativity, pollution can all throw its delicate mechanism out of sync. If the cause is not treated, the imbalance will spread and eventually the physical, material, skin and bones body will suffer. However, treat the subtle energy of the body, and quite incredible things can happen.

There are now hundreds of different forms of energy medicine – from acupuncture to zero balancing. They are all worth investigating and trying for yourself. But, for the purposes of this book, I want to look at just a few that you can easily and readily use yourself.

SHIATSU – FINGER PRESSURE FOR SIMPLE HEALING

In Japanese, shiatsu combines two words: shi (finger) + atsu (pressure), literally, finger pressure. But shiatsu is not massage. The philosophy is different and so is the touch. Obviously, to enjoy the full benefits of shiatsu you would need to find an experienced and qualified shiatsu practitioner: however, there is a lot we can do for ourselves. We all practise an instinctive form of self-shiatsu every time we press our foreheads to relieve a headache, or pinch the bridge of our noses to ease eye strain, or rub our arms briskly when we feel cold.

First steps in Shiatsu

The pressure you use in those instinctive exercises should be a guide when you practise some of the techniques given here. There's a subtle art in applying pressure slowly and evenly to avoid pain and resistance. Practise on yourself first before you practise on others. Press down slowly, hold to a count of five and release slowly. Don't make the common mistake of thinking you have to wiggle your thumb or make rapid circular movements to be effective. You don't. You just press in and hold.

Some people prefer a light pressure. Others can take quite a deep pressure. You will soon find out what works best for you. Shiatsu is a peaceful and concentrated technique, as you will discover the more you practise it.

exercise

Try this simple exercise. Inhale and exhale slowly. Raise your hands, palms facing one another. Gradually move them together and apart, without touching. Move in slow motion. Keep your eyes closed if this helps you concentrate. In time you may feel a magnetic pull between your palms. That is your energetic force and it will grow the more you do this exercise. Now, find a tense or tight muscle on your leg. Place your hands on it and feel the warmth. Then place your thumb on it and press down gradually. Don't jab. Don't be in a hurry. The slower you press, the deeper you can go. Hold the point, count to five. Release slowly. Repeat the exercise a couple of times. Now, move an inch or so along the tight muscle and try again. Move on another inch, and try again.
With practise you may feel increasing warmth, tingling, a release of tension or pain.

As you might have guessed, what you are doing when you press in this way is stimulating or releasing blocked ki (which equates to chi in Chinese) – vital energy or life force.

Our bodies are always striving towards health: illness is simply the body's way of telling us that something is wrong on a more subtle level

exercise

Self-healing with Shiatsu

Self-shiatsu can help us deal better with many of the problems of modern life. Try practising the following routines to feel the difference balancing your vital energy will make to everyday life.

STRESSBUSTING

Stress can be our worst enemy. We all suffer from it, or from stress-related aches and pains. Here's a simple series of exercises to help combat stress.

1. Hunch and drop your shoulders a couple of times, then rotate them to ease that 'tortoise' syndrome of hunched shoulders and a compressed neck.

2. Sit for a moment, close your eyes and breathe deeply.

3. Look up and stretch your arms, reaching for the sky, first with one hand, then the other.

4. Rub your head briskly. Tap it all over with your fingertips. Tug your hair then swiftly release your hands.

5. Squeeze around your jaw-line and tap your jaw-line (particularly good for jaw clenchers and teeth grinders.)

6. Clench your jaw. Open your mouth wide, imagining you are an opera singer and say 'Aaaaaaah'!

7. Squeeze your eyes shut and open them wide. Repeat.

8. Close your eyes while you inhale and exhale slowly, concentrating on the flow of air through your nostrils. If you can, picture something peaceful and beautiful, a flower, a line of poetry, the face of a loved one.

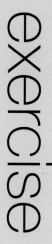

BANISHING HEADACHES

Blocked energy through the neck and shoulders can lead to headaches. Use these techniques on a daily basis if you are prone to headaches – they work best as a preventative measure. Press the points to the count of five, release slowly, press again, release. Repeat a few times.

1. Press the inside corners of each eye. You'll find the points if you pinch the bridge of your nose.

2. Press points under your eyebrows. Rest your head on your fingertips if necessary.

3. Pinch your eyebrows.

4. Fingers apart, grip your head and work along parallel and diagonal lines extending over the top of your head and down your neck.

5. Draw soft circles on your temples (without pressure).

6. Anchor your thumbs under your occipital ridge – just behind your ears on your hairline. Tilt your head forward and back.

7. Squeeze the back of your neck.

8. Bunch your fists against your sacrum (lower back) and lean back (or lie down on the floor and place a tennis ball under your sacrum).

9. Pinch your little toe (and your big toe).

SOOTHING INSOMNIA

If counting sheep doesn't help you and you are weary of making yourself hot drinks with honey, watching TV, listening to music, reading etc. you could try some of the following exercises.

1. Lie on your back. Slide your fingers under your neck and apply gentle pressure.

2. Practice deep breathing. Imagine your breath as a silver stream entering your left nostril, sitting at the top of your nose as you hold your breath to a count of five, and exiting your right nostril. Repeat.

3. Tighten your entire body, from the tips of your toes to your scalp. Release each part in turn.

exercise

BANISHING THE BLUES – BOOSTING ENERGY

'Pebble therapy' is a great way to beat the blues and pick up your energy levels when you're feeling down. It is also good for poor circulation, or for stiff joints.

1. Take a handful of pebbles, roll them around in your palm and squeeze them. Open and close your hand several times. Now squeeze the pebbles between your fingers.

2. Press your bare feet on them, roll the pebbles around the floor underfoot and try picking them up between your toes.

HEALING

Once you've felt energy moving in your body through shiatsu, you are ready to go one step further. Let's look now at hands-off healing! Pure spiritual healing is perhaps the ultimate energyworking tool, and it's something we can all do. Some of us might be healing every day – without even realizing. A mother rocking her baby sends healing energy to soothe and make the infant feel secure. A loving squeeze of the hand sends a boost of reassuring energy to a child heading off for a tough day at school. A cool hand across a fevered forehead can help the healing process when someone is sick. Even total strangers can give the healing touch: some people simply shake your hand or put a hand on your shoulder and you can almost feel their energy leaping out at you.

Healing seems so simple – the healer either just touches the person or hovers their hands above him or her. Some use specific holds and imagine certain symbols, as in Reiki, the Japanese form of healing. Some simply sit and think about their patient getting well, even though they are miles apart. So how can it work? Many healers believe they are channeling a higher form of energy, from God or some spiritual source. Others are more prosaic and simply say they are balancing the person's own energy system. Many healers insist they do not actively heal but merely open up the body so it can perform its own healing.

The first step to becoming a healer is to be able to sense subtle energy. You can probably already do this if you have followed the exercises in this book. Now you need to be able to focus it through your hands. This is actually incredibly simple – just the next step on from the first shiatsu exercise.

AWAKENING YOUR HANDS

1. Rub your hands together quite vigorously for a few moments.

2. Now hold them a few inches apart, as you did in the shiatsu exercise. But this time imagine you are holding a ball. You may feel a tingling or a warmth from your hands. 'Bounce ' your hands and feel the energy change as your hands move closer and further away.

3. Take your hands even further apart, as if you were holding, say, a football.

4. Now imagine that in the centre of your palm is a circular patch which can transmit energy. Rub this area with the thumb of your other hand, imagining you are opening up this area. Then repeat on the other hand. If you have any religious or spiritual belief you could ask for help in your healing quest.

CHANNELLING HEALING ENERGY

1. Stand in a relaxed position, as we have done with all the exercises in this book. Breathe slowly and deeply for a few minutes to centre yourself.

2. Once again, imagine your chakras open and spinning in perfect harmony. In particular remember to ground yourself by opening the base chakra.

3. Now imagine you are pulling down vital energy through your crown chakra. The energy shoots through your body, linking up all the chakras. Spend a few moments allowing the energy to settle to a comfortable level.

4. Breathe in the energy and pull it to your heart chakra. Think about what you want to achieve with this healing energy; ask permission to become a channel for this healing.

5. From the heart chakra, imagine the energy shooting out along your arms to your hands. It tingles and buzzes in your hands, rippling along your fingers.

6. Now direct the energy to wherever you want it to go (either to a part of your own body or to someone else).

exercise

exercise

HEALING SOMEONE ELSE

1. Work through the previous exercise. While you are doing this, ask the person you wish to heal to either stand, sit or lie comfortably. Ask them to just relax, close their eyes and breathe naturally.

2. When you feel the energy coursing through your fingers you can direct the healing energy to them. If you know a particular area is causing problems, simply hold your hands on or over that area. Visualize the healing energy streaming into that spot.

3. If you want to do a more general healing, simply let your hands move as they wish. You may feel drawn to touch a particular part of the body – or not to touch the body at all but to keep your hands a few inches away. Let your intuition guide you. If you like you could focus on each of the chakras, visualizing your energy balancing each of them.

4. As you work, you might feel your hands become stiff or uncomfortable. Quietly shake them to release any negative energy you might have picked up while working.

ENERGY GAMES

The best way to learn about healing energy is to use it, practice it, play with it. Don't be scared of it – it is as natural as breathing! It can also be great fun – so let yourself go and enjoy it. If you can, enlist the help of a partner and try these exercises.

● Number One aims to direct energy to the other while Number Two tries to resist it. It can be remarkably hard to resist receiving energy. If you are the person trying to give energy how could you sneak past the other person's defenses? If you are the person resisting, how could you protect yourself? These are useful techniques as we will discover in later chapters. Sometimes it can be very useful to avoid energy!

● Number One closes their eyes while Number Two directs energy to a particular part of the body. Number One has to guess where the energy is being directed.

● Number One lies down while Number Two scans their energy field. With your hands four or five inches above their body, run your hands from the top of the head down to the feet. Can you feel any areas of imbalance? What do you notice? Do any parts feel hot? Cold? Congested? What does your intuition tell you? Remember you are not diagnosing but sensing. Ask Number One if they have any discomfort or problems in the areas you picked up.

● If someone has a pain or problem, you can try to 'draw off' the pain through your hands. Simply hold your hands over the spot and imagine the negative energy coming up into your hands. As you feel it in your hands, gently shake it away, imagining it being absorbed and transformed into pure energy.

TAKING HEALING FURTHER

Once you have come to grips with the basic principles of healing, there are plenty of other techniques and 'props' you can use to extend your healing repertoire. Experiment to see which suit you and which have the best effects. We are all very different and it really is a case of horses for courses.

We can all heal –
it's a skill that can be learned like any other

HOMEOPATHY AND FLOWER ESSENCES

Homeopathy has always infuriated orthodox medicine. How could it possibly work when there is not even one molecule of its original substance left? Yet now researchers are beginning to unravel the mysteries of homeopathy, paving the way for a greater understanding of subtle energy medicine in general. It seems as though the water in which the remedies are diluted can extract and store a memory of the subtle energy of the healing substance, which, in turn, affects the subtle energy of the body. Hahnemann, who founded homeopathy, believed that the remedies were working very much like a classic immunization, by creating an artificial illness in the patient that has very similar characteristics to the illness the physician wants to remove. The artificial illness stimulates the body's natural defenses, which then rise up to cure the original ailment. It seems, however, that the remedy, rather than producing a physical reaction at a structural cell level, is producing a vibrational reaction, a vibrational illness to stimulate the body to heal at a vibrational level. You can learn to use homeopathy yourself for first aid purposes, although to use it at its most powerful you would need a full four or five year training. So I would recommend that the novice energyworker start with flower essences.

He thought the essences worked on an energetic level, invigorating and balancing the psyche.

Flower (and gem) essences seem to work on a similar vibrational level to homeopathy – although they predominantly work on emotional, rather than physical problems. Dr Edward Bach, who discovered the original Bach Flower Essences in Britain, became convinced by homeopathy – he didn't think it was necessary to ingest the whole crude plant (as in herbalism or orthodox medicine), but to take in the essence of the plant. He thought the essences worked on an energetic level, invigorating and balancing the psyche.

I absolutely love the Bach flower remedies and have used them for the past 20 years or so. They are totally safe to use – even on babies and animals – and really do bring about change. If you want an introduction to energy healing, this is a great place to start. Simply choose the remedy or remedies (any number up to six or seven) that suit your current mood and add two drops of each to a 30ml 'stock ' bottle of fresh spring water. Then take four drops four times daily – directly into your mouth or added to your glass of water or cup of coffee.

The Bach flower remedies

These are the main personality traits associated with the 38 remedies.

FOR FEAR: Aspen (vague, undefined fears that something is wrong, supernatural fears); Mimulus (fear of known things – heights, spiders, meeting people etc); Cherry Plum (irrational thoughts and fears, fear of loss of control, violent temper); Red Chestnut (over-anxiety and fear for others); Rock Rose (sheer terror, sudden shocks and alarm).

FOR UNCERTAINTY: Cerato (doubting your self-judgment); Gorse (hopelessness, pessimism); Gentian (despondency, discouragement); Hornbeam (lack of energy, listlessness); Scleranthus (indecisiveness, fluctuating moods), Wild Oat (lack of direction in life, uncertainty about career – very useful for teenagers and students).

FOR LONELINESS: Impatiens (impatience, irritable, intolerant); Heather (self-obsessed, hates to be alone), Water Violet (aloofness, disdain, seems remote).

FOR OVER-SENSITIVITY: Agrimony (torturing thoughts hidden behind cheerful facade); Centaury (timidity, subservience); Holly (envy, jealousy, hatred); Walnut (difficulty adapting to change, good for rites of passage, e.g. puberty, menopause; or for shifts in circumstance – e.g. moving, new job).

FOR DESPONDENCY OR DESPAIR: Crab Apple (self-disgust, hates body, feels unclean or ashamed); Elm (normally copes well but overwhelmed by responsibility); Larch (lack of confidence, gives up easily); Oak (brave, determined, struggling on against the odds); Pine (guilt, self-blame), Sweet Chestnut (extreme despair); Star of Bethlehem (for after-effects of severe shock); Willow (resentment, bitterness, self-pitying).

FOR OVERCONCERN FOR OTHERS: Beech (intolerant, critical, has to be right); Chicory (selfishness, possessiveness); Vervain (over-enthusiastic, fanatical); Vine (domineering); Rock Water (self-repression).

FOR INSUFFICIENT INTEREST IN THE PRESENT: Chestnut Bud (keeps repeating same mistakes); Clematis (daydreaming); Honeysuckle (nostalgia, lives in the past – often good for old people); Mustard (depression); Olive (exhaustion, 'burn-out '); White Chestnut (persistent worries); Wild Rose (resignation, apathy).

SOUND THERAPY

We've already experienced a taster of sound therapy, in our chakra toning exercises. It's a form of subtle energy healing which is as old as time. Apparently the ancient esoteric schools of India and Tibet, Greece and Egypt all taught the importance of the power of sound: vibration was held to be the basic creative force of the universe. The Bible says exactly that: 'In the beginning was the Word.' And the Qabalah places precise and great importance on sounds. Simply making different sounds can affect your whole mood. If you're feeling tired, take a few moments and simply groan – really loudly and with complete abandon. Slump down, let your arms flop by your sides and groan as loud as you can. Sound healer Chris James reckons this is one of the best ways to release any negative emotions – and it works!

'Disease is simply part of our bodies vibrating out of tune,' says pioneering sound therapist Jonathan Goldman.

If you're feeling tense, try softly humming to yourself. This soothing sound seems to calm the brain. If you listen to young babies, one of the first sounds they make is a soft 'mmmm' which they tend to repeat over and over when they feel uncertain or unhappy – it appears to comfort them.

'Disease is simply part of our bodies vibrating out of tune,' says pioneering sound therapist Jonathan Goldman. 'Every organ, bone, tissue and other part of the body has a healthy resonant frequency. When that frequency alters, that part of the body vibrates out of harmony and that is what is termed disease. If it were possible to determine the correct resonant frequency for a healthy organ and then project it into that part which is diseased, the organ should return to its normal frequency and a healing should occur.'

Goldman firmly believes that, by creating sounds that are harmonious with the 'correct frequency of the healthy organ, we could all learn how to heal ourselves, bringing our bodies back into balance. He, along with other sound researchers, have been focusing most of their attention on the sacred chants of varying traditions, believing that the high-frequency harmonics that most of them share, could be having profound effects on both the mind and body.

Take time to practise the chakra toning exercise as often as you can – it is a powerful exercise in sound therapy.

COLOUR THERAPY

Can colour change your life? Researchers into the incredible world of colour have found that the colours that surround us – in our homes and workplaces, in the clothes we wear and even the foods we eat – can have enormous effects on our life. Colour can affect everything from health to happiness, from success to our sex lives. Red walls in a pub could mean more fights at closing time. Pink walls in a prison, on the other hand, make inmates quieter and less aggressive.

Colour therapists, meanwhile, use 'chromatotherapy', lamps with different coloured filters that flood the body with colour; some prescribe 'colour diets' or advise clients to dress in certain colours or decorate their houses in particular hues to heal both physical and emotional conditions. Practitioners of colourpuncture beam combinations of colour onto specific points of the body to achieve seemingly miraculous cures – for everything from migraine to bronchitis. It sounds far-fetched, but a growing band of solid scientific research seems to back up the claims. Carlton Wagner, director of the Wagner Institute for Color Research in California, has shown that viewing certain colours evokes physical change. David Rainey, Ph.D. of John Carroll University in Ohio, agrees. He has found that seeing red can stimulate the glandular system and increase the heart rate, blood pressure and respiration.

One of the best known experiments in the use of colour showed that patients with high blood pressure could lower their blood pressure on demand simply by visualizing the colour blue. When they visualized red, the blood pressure rose. Colour therapists weren't remotely surprised.

Helen Irlen, a psychologist from California, has discovered that adult students with reading difficulties can often be helped by using coloured filters. And colour researcher Marie Louise Lacy also cites research into the effects of colour on severely handicapped children and children with learning difficulties.

In the meantime, dose yourself with as broad a spectrum of colour as possible. If your problems involve coldness, poor circulation, lethargy, constipation you need to invoke the warmer colours – reds, oranges, yellows and pinks. In fact, research in America showed that painting your bathroom in warm oranges and reds could actually help to cure constipation! On the other hand, if you are feverish or suffer from inflammation and 'hot' conditions, then the soothing blue and green shades could quite literally cool you down.

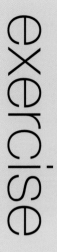

COLOUR BREATHING

This exercise can be very healing. Do it for yourself when you are feeling under par or direct someone else through the exercise.

1. Lie down and make yourself comfortable.

2. Choose a colour from those below that suits your problem.

3. Visualize the colour as a cloud that you can slowly inhale through the pores of your skin. The coloured cloud comes in your body through your fingers and toes and then travels through your body (visualize your bones as hollow so the colour can seep through).

4. Then, as you exhale, imagine the colour leaving your body, taking with it all the sickness, the toxins, the illness. It all leaves your body and harmlessly vapourizes.

5. Repeat several times.

Colour correspondences

Red: good for circulation, problems with the blood, sexual problems, ill-effects of cold, numbness.

Orange: helps depression, hernias, kidney stones. Can help milk flow in breastfeeding mothers.

Yellow: good for indigestion, constipation. Supports the lymphatic system, diabetes, kidneys and liver.

Green: good for nervous conditions, colds, flu, ulcers, hay fever.

Turquoise: helps throat problems, anti-inflammatory

Blue: excellent for pain relief, for bleeding and burns, colic, respiratory problems, skin problems and rheumatism.

Indigo: helps migraine, soothes ear and eye problems, skin disorders, nervous system.

Violet: emotional problems, arthritis, can ease childbirth

Magenta: good for heart and mental problems.

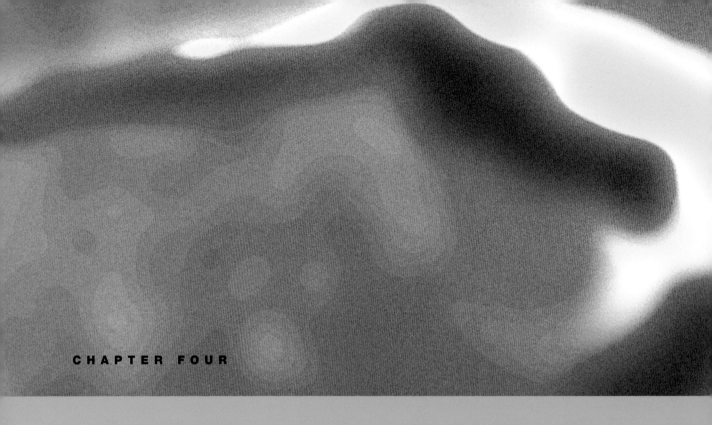

CHAPTER FOUR

THE ENERGETIC POWER OF FOOD

Without food we have no energy. Without food, we have no life at all. So why do so many of us take so little care over the nutrition we give our bodies? If you want to cultivate vital energy in your life, you have to look at what you eat. But don't panic – this isn't going to be a chapter insisting you follow some spartan hair-shirt diet, it's about the totally fascinating alchemy of food. The energy of food is partly about the actual foods we choose to eat, but it also goes way beyond eggs and bacon, lentils and tofu. It's about how we cook our food, how we eat our food, how we think about food. It's not just about which foods are good for our bodies (although that is important), but about which foods are good for our minds, emotions, and even our spiritual well-being.

Let's start our hunt for this spirit and soul food in the ancient cultures of India and China...

THE SATTVIC DIET – THE AYURVEDIC WAY OF FOOD

'Prana is the life force of the universe,' says Deepak Chopra, 'and it goes into you, in me, with food.' In Ayurveda, great care is taken over the foods that are eaten. Ayurveda teaches that a subtle energy substance, called ojas, is extracted from food once it has been perfectly digested (note the perfectly!) Ojas imbues our cells with energy or, as Chopra puts it, 'Enables the cells to "feel happy", to experience the cellular equivalent of bliss.'

It sounds good but how can we maximize the amount of ojas extracted from our food? The answer lies in what the ayurvedic physicians call the 'sattvic diet'. Basically Ayurveda classes all foodstuffs as either sattvic, rajasic or tamasic. Sattvic foods are considered to promote life, health, happiness and satisfaction. They help us become serene and contented – they balance our energies. Rajassic foods are powerful, pungent, sour, harsh and burning – they tend to make our energy overactive and aggressive. Tamasic foods are 'dead' foods – tasteless, stale, leftover or overly-processed. They make our energy become stagnant, sluggish, lazy, inert. Put like this you'd imagine we'd all be clamouring to eat sattvic food but sadly it's not the case. How many of us live on a high-stress diet of coffee, alcohol and seering hot takeaways? How many of us 'make time' by shoving another ready-meal in the microwave or shovelling down a stale cake or leftovers from the fridge?

Ayurveda has been practised for well over 5,000 years and the ancient sages learned through painstaking observation how different foods reacted with their bodies, minds and spirits. Their highly trained senses could detect the vibrational effects of each and every food. They noted that an apple growing on a tree has a quite different energy from that same apple once picked. Once it was cooked, it changed again. In our crazy world we would never give ourselves the time to come to such awareness, but we can at least follow their advice based on millennia of wisdom.

Sattvic foods
Generally sattvic foods are:

● light, soothing and easily digested

● fresh – as fresh as possible – seasonal, grown locally and organically

● moderate in portion size.

The most sattvic foods are all sweet in nature and include milk, ghee (clarified butter), fruits and fruit juices, sesame seeds, rice, honey, wheat, mung beans, coconut, dates and spring water. Some of these sound strange at first reading. Milk, after all, can be very mucous-forming. Ayurveda has an answer to that: milk should always be boiled before drinking – it makes it more digestible. If you still find it indigestible, add a pinch of dried ginger or turmeric before boiling. The sattvic diet, it must be remembered, is designed for people who spend a lot of time being serene or aiming at serenity! In other words meditating, doing yoga, contemplating and generally not having to get by in a stressed world. Obviously you might say there are times when this kind of diet doesn't pass muster – you need some of those rajassic foods to buck you up and get you through the day. Well, fair enough (in fact as we'll see the Chinese system is more even-handed when it comes to looking at these high-energy foods). But, while you can't base your entire diet around these foods, think of trying them when you need the ultimate comfort foods – calming and highly soothing. And there is absolutely no excuse for eating tamasic foods – at least I can't think of one!

Ayurveda also teaches the importance of how you eat. Although food should always taste good, it also needs to attract the other senses. So make sure your plate looks attractive – and your table as well. Can you be really inventive and find foods that sound good – or that feel good in the mouth? Think about texture – the soft hairiness of a peach, the smooth sensation of yogurt, the crisp bite of stir-fried vegetables.

THE AYURVEDIC RULES FOR GOOD ENERGY EATING

Ayurveda has very strict rules for good eating. If you follow these you will undoubtedly give your body the best chance of absorbing ojas, and enjoying ultimate energetic balance.

● Make mealtimes a time of settled, calm pleasure. Never eat when you are upset or angry.

● Always sit down to eat. Set aside a decent time to eat and concentrate purely on your eating. Eat at a moderate pace – neither wolfing it down nor dawdling for too long.

● By all means have pleasant company while eating but don't talk while you are chewing your food.

● Wherever possible ensure your food is freshly cooked – use fresh, local, organic produce in season wherever possible. Avoid at all costs stale, processed, convenience and junk food.

● Avoid ice-cold food and drink. Minimize the amount of raw food you eat – it is harder to digest. Drink only warm water with your meals (some physicians advise you don't drink at all with meals as it interferes with the digestive process). If you like to drink milk, don't have it with meals – drink it separately.

● Don't eat unless you are hungry. And don't stuff yourself until you are full. Always leave around a third or a quarter of your stomach empty to help your digestion.

● If possible incorporate all the six tastes into your meals – these are sweet (i.e. milk, butter, rice, bread, pasta), sour (yogurt, cheese, lemon, vinegar), salty (salt, tamari, soy sauce), pungent (ginger, onions, hot peppers, cumin), bitter (green leafy vegetables, turmeric), astringent (beans, lentils).

● Don't race up after a meal – sit quietly for a few minutes and give thanks.

THE TAO OF EATING

Like Ayurveda, Chinese traditional medicine (TCM) teaches the importance of good eating for optimum energy. Food is so important that many traditional physicians will try to cure illness using food alone. Only if the disease is very resistant will they move on to use herbs or, as a last resort, acupuncture. Good food is considered good medicine and, as with all Chinese therapy, the aim is to achieve an optimum balance of energy.

If you are feeling fine and in balance, you can keep that way by observing the external environment and adapting your diet to balance that.

As in Ayurveda, food is considered to release a vital essence – it is specifically seen as an alchemical act, essential nutrients being transformed into energy. Where Ayurveda breaks foods down into sattvic, rajastic and tamasic, Chinese philosophy predominantly breaks food down into yin and yang and considers both useful. Yin foods are generally calming and cooling in their effects (like sattvic foods) while yang foods are warming and stimulating (more akin to rajastic). Like Ayurveda, TCM frowns on rotten, left-over, tired and processed foods.

So it makes sense that if your own energy is low and deficient, if you were feeling depressed, tired or sluggish, you would try to boost it with yang foods while if you are stressed, over-excited and angry you would need the soothing effects of yin foods. If you are feeling fine and in balance, you can keep that way by observing the external environment and adapting your diet to balance that. So if it were cold, overcast and damp you should aim for a mainly yang diet. If it's very hot and dry, go for a yin diet.

YIN FOODS COOLING – ALKALINE-FORMING	YANG FOODS WARMING – ACID-FORMING
raw fruits and vegetables	cooked fruits and vegetables
salads	dried and stewed fruit
rice, bulgur	lentils, kidney beans
milk, yogurt	potatoes, root vegetables
bean sprouts, tofu	oats, barley
sugar, salt	meat and cooked fish
soy sauce, tamari, seaweed	nuts and seeds
chilli peppers, curry powder (surprising but true!)	garlic, ginger, black pepper, cloves
parsley, coriander	basil, thyme, oregano, bay leaf
raw fish (sushi)	chocolate, vanilla
	miso, molasses

Daniel Reid, author of several books on the Tao, has studied the art of eating in great detail and believes that the key to the energy exchange in food lies with the enzymes of the body. 'Enzymes are endowed with a spark of living energy, or chi, and it is this energy which gives them their remarkable bioactive powers,' he says. He goes on to warn that our modern eating habits do nothing to help enzyme activity. 'Modern farming, food-processing and cooking methods produce foods that are completely enzyme-dead. Such diets slowly but surely deplete vitality and therefore shorten life. Only wholesome natural foods consumed in a relatively natural state produce wholesome natural energy for the body.'

SPIRIT AND SOUL FOOD

Having looked briefly at what constitutes a healthy diet, let's look at something much more esoteric – how the very way we cook and even eat our food can affect its vital energy. Does it really matter if we lovingly chop our vegetables by hand, or simply chuck them in the food processor? Can it really make a difference whether we sit down, say a prayer and mindfully eat our food or whether we chomp it down while we watch TV or munch as we drive along the highway? Apparently so.

Among other cultures, culinary art is also an art of life. The Sufis, for instance, hold that our health, happiness, liberty and judgment are all affected by what happens in our kitchens.

This idea would, of course, be of no surprise to the ancient Ayurvedic and Chinese sages. Nor to virtually every ancient culture in the world. Carrie L'Esperance, writing in *The Ancient Cookfire*, says 'Thousands of years ago, people realized that not only body structure but even human nature can be changed by attending to the manner in which we eat and drink. For these ancients, eating and drinking were considered the most important rituals in the divine art of life. Among other cultures, culinary art is also an art of life. The Sufis, for instance, hold that our health, happiness, liberty and judgment are all affected by what happens in our kitchens.'

Deborah Kesten, a nutritionist and author of *Feeding the Body, Nourishing the Soul*, agrees. She is concerned that in our frantic modern-day society, food has been reduced to 'fuel' and that we are concerned with nothing other than its basic nutritional value. The ultimate symbol of this 'eat it fast' mentality is the drive-thru diner – at some gas stations you can even order your hamburger while you fill your tank! But, as she points out, the human body is not a machine and many of the food-related issues that plague us – from overeating to anorexia – can be traced to our lack of awareness of the relationship between body and soul. She firmly believes that our problems with food come about because we have lost our spiritual connection to the food we eat. We have lost the energetic link.

Almost every spiritual tradition, from the Sufi to the Native American, from the Jewish to the Christian, from the Hindu to the Muslim regards food as sacred – and the eating of food as a sacrament

Her theory is backed up by research in the US – scientists are finding that how food is prepared can actually affect its nutritional content and taste. Other researchers are convinced that the way we eat our food and the attitude we bring to it, can make a difference to how it is metabolized. 'Is it possible that food may receive, store and 'give back' to us the energy and consciousness that we give to our food?' asks Kesten. The answer seems to be yes. She insists this is not as farfetched as it seems and points to ancient wisdom traditions – from Judaism to Hinduism, from Christianity to Native American shamanism – all of which imbue food with spirit. 'Enlightened eating acknowledges the inherent sacred quality of food,' says Kesten, 'that it is life-filled and life-giving, offering biological, psychological and spiritual sustenance.'

Projecting loving energy to an orange actually changed the taste and texture of the fruit – it peeled more easily and was juicier and sweeter. 'Spiritually imbued' cheap wine took on the taste of a classic vintage.

In the scientific community, the link between consciousness and food is still in the early stages of exploration. Dr. Larry Dossey, a scientist investigating the link between science and spirituality says, 'That our consciousness affects matter (including food) is not in doubt. HOW it happens is a huge mystery.'

Physicist Fred Alan Wolf Ph.D., says it is insufficient to ask, 'What nutrients are in the food?' Rather, we should be asking 'What were you thinking about when you were eating?' A new scientific field is in the making – one that may give us a prescription for creating an as yet unidentified 'nutrient' that manifests through the wisdom and awareness we bring to our food. Maybe this is the ojas of Ayurveda? Numerous experiments have shown that healing can increase the energy and growing capacity of seeds and can even keep milk fresh longer. Dr. Laskow, a leading researcher in the field discovered that by combining intention, visualization and healing energy, food could be transformed – it could literally contain more vitality, more healing powers. Projecting loving energy to an orange actually changed the taste and texture of the fruit – it peeled more easily and was juicier and sweeter. 'Spiritually imbued' cheap wine took on the taste of a classic vintage.

Try the following to test whether you can detect the energetic difference between 'ordinary' food and food imbued with spiritual energy.

● Processed v hand-prepared vegetables. Make a salad – chop half of the vegetables by hand, using a knife and cutting board; chop the other half in a food processor. Can you detect the difference?

● Cooking consciously v unconsciously. Before enjoying a favourite dish, shop for, prepare, cook and eat the food with a loving consciousness. As a contrast, next time you prepare the same dish, choose to do so during an especially busy time – so do everything in a hurry, without any care or thought. Can you detect any difference?

exercise

CREATING FOOD WITH LOVING ENERGY
Here's how to infuse food and liquids with loving, spiritual energy.

1. Sit or stand in a comfortable position. Become aware of your breathing. Consciously relax your body. Breathe more deeply.

2. Focus your attention on your heart chakra, imagining you are breathing in and out through that area. Activate the heart chakra by thinking of people you love, a wonderful moment in your life – anything which brings up loving, caring feelings.

3. Now visualize a shimmering sphere of light several inches above your head, the crown chakra. The powerful energy from this sphere comes down into your head and descends through the chakras into your heart and hands.

4. Now remind yourself that you can project this healing, wonderful energy into the food or drink before you. The light comes out through your heart and hands and soaks into the food. Surround both sides of the dish with your hands and feel the energy emanating from both of your hands, pouring into the food or drink.

exercise

EATING MEDITATION

Jon Kabat-Zinn, Ph.D., of the Stress Reduction Clinic at the University of Massachusetts Medical Center, suggests practising mindfulness meditation while you eat, to foster the correct relationship between your mind and your food.

1. Look at a piece of food – say a raisin. Imagine you are a Martian scientist who has come to earth and never seen one before. What do you see?

2. Bring it to your nose and smell it. How does it smell, what is its scent?

3. Now notice what is going on in your mouth – the physiological reaction to the raisin. You might be salivating – even though the raisin is not in your mouth yet. This is the mind/body phenomenon – you are reacting to the anticipation of the food.

4. Now explore how the raisin feels.

5. Think about how your hand will bring the raisin to your lips. How does your hand know how to deliver the raisin to your mouth? Be aware of this motion as you bring the raisin up to and into your mouth. What does your tongue do with the raisin? How does it get it between your teeth? Become conscious of the normally unconscious act of chewing.

6. Bite into the raisin consciously, slowly. Start to chew. Notice what is happening in your mouth. How does it taste? There are hundreds of words to describe taste – really think about it.

7. As you chew, the taste changes. So does the consistency. What is the texture of the raisin?

8. Don't swallow yet, even though you might be starting to feel an aversion to the raisin in your mouth. Become aware of the aversion. Then swallow, following the path of the raisin to the back of your mouth. Then in your mind's eye follow it down into the stomach. Become aware that you are now one raisin heavier.

If you follow this meditation with all your meals your relationship to food will totally change.

SOUL SHOPPING AND SPIRITUAL COOKERY

As we've seen, there is far more to food than calories. Yes, food provides us with the basic energy we need to keep going, but it does far more than that. By acknowledging that our food contains subtle energy which can be protected or destroyed by the way we prepare and eat it, we should start to look at buying, cooking and eating food in a totally new way.

Think about where the food has come from – imagine it in its original surroundings: orange juice from the sun-kissed orange groves; cereal from the glistening rows of wheat and corn; bacon from pigs rooting around (hopefully in open fields and woodland).

As the most energetically pure food is fresh, seasonal and organic, why not think about growing (at least some of) your own food? You don't need a huge garden – you could at the very least have a window box of culinary herbs (which smell nice too and help keep the bugs away) or put a few grow-bags with tomatoes or peas on your porch or balcony. Lettuces grow quite happily in hanging baskets, beans will clamber up a wall with the help of some trellis. If you can't grow your own, try to buy your food from local suppliers (maybe even direct from the farm?) OK, so that's impossible – you live in the heart of a great big city. Well, join an organic box scheme so you can support people who are trying to grow food as naturally as possible. Insist on organic produce and try to buy food that is in season.

Above all, think about your shopping – whether you live in the heart of the country or the hub of the city. Try if you can to buy food as and when you need it, rather than doing a huge shop each week and stuffing most of it in the freezer. Make mealtimes something special. Treat yourself to some really attractive cookbooks and take time deciding what you would like to cook and eat. Make a list of what you need and try to find time to source the best possible ingredients available. Be conscious as you choose your produce – pick each vegetable with awareness. Notice its shape. Think about where the food has come from – imagine it in its original surroundings (orange juice from the sun-kissed orange groves; cereal from the glistening rows of wheat and corn; bacon from pigs rooting around (hopefully in open fields and woodland).

All too often we don't consider the origins of our food. We abnegate responsibility – we accept food that has been genetically modified and irradiated, stuffed full of preservatives, pesticides and hormones. When you start to think where your food comes from you may find your eating habits totally change. Which would you prefer: eggs from hens that roam free, scratching in fields as nature planned or eggs from hens that have 'lived' their lives in tiny cramped hutches, barely able to move? Which egg do you think would have the best energy? Which would convert most easily to ojas in your body? Go a step further: who created the mass-produced soup in the can? Did they lovingly slice the vegetables, chop the herbs with care, stir the soup with love and awareness? Unlikely, isn't it? So how about making your own 'soul' soup – preparing each ingredient with mindfulness and imbuing the dish with love as you prepare it. You might say a prayer for each person who will eat it, imagining that you are cooking a magical pot with healing powers. 'This is for my dear friend who is battling with depression, every stir of the spoon endows this meal with vital energy and joy and hope. As she eats it she will feel the life return to her body, mind and soul.' You could bake 'conception cookies for someone trying to conceive but having difficulty. 'Love' porridge to catch the heart of the person you want to attract. Fanciful? Remember that research into how our thoughts and prayers can affect food? Just try it.

Which would you prefer: eggs from hens that roam free, scratching in fields as nature planned or eggs from hens that have 'lived' their lives in tiny cramped hutches, barely able to move? Which egg do you think would have the best energy?

If you start to look on cookery as a kind of spell-making, you can boost your magic-making powers with the use of herbs and spices. Check out two wonderful novels for inspiration, *Like Water for Chocolate* by Laura Esquival is a feast of a novel, describing how consciously created meals produced dramatic effects! *Mistress of Spices* by Chitra Banerjee Divakaruni is another magical read – about the magical powers of spices and how they altered lives.

But on a practical note, here are some of the less well-known attributes of common herbs and spices:

● **mint:** the great cleanser, use it when you or people around you have been sick or been around 'negative' people or places. Note: use peppermint with caution if breastfeeding – it can reduce milk flow.

● **rosemary:** a protective plant – use it when you are feeling unsure, nervous or scared. It is also the herb of remembrance.

● **parsley:** another protector – against negative energy. Use it if you're feeling a bit down or 'got at' by people at work or nasty neighbours!

● **sage:** the wisdom plant, as the name suggests. Use it when you feel you need more wisdom or to learn some lesson of life. Note: if you suffer from epilepsy, avoid sage (it can trigger seizures) – if you are pregnant only add very small amounts to cooking – don't take it in medicinal doses.

● **dill:** linked with prosperity, drop some in the pot when finances are tight and you might get a nice surprise.

● **lemon balm:** a plant of healing and achievement. Use it when anyone has been or is sick – or perhaps when children are going in for exams. It is also said to 'comfort the heart and drive away sadness'.

● **nutmeg:** said to induce romance and healing. But use with caution – a pinch is enough.

● **saffron:** said by the ancients to imbue those who eat it with youth and life-force. It is also very welcoming to guests.

● **ginger:** used in ancient cultures to communicate with the gods. Use in a cooking 'prayer' sending your hopes and wishes to heaven with its scent. Note: use with caution during pregnancy; avoid if you suffer from excess acidity or peptic ulcers.

● **turmeric:** a good luck spice, use for special meals before exams or moving house, or weddings. Supposedly particularly beneficial for babies – so use in christening meals – and anoint the baby's head with a tiny bit of turmeric like a bindi.

MAKE MEALTIMES SPECIAL

In days gone by mealtimes were a time of gathering, when families and extended family and friends gathered together. They were a time of discussion, of sharing stories, of giving advice and sympathy, of laughter and sometimes tears. Now we rarely eat together and we miss out on the communal energy of the shared table. Very simple things can make mealtimes special:

Think about the appearance of your meals and lay your table with great care and attention. Polish the wood, or lay a pretty cloth. It needn't be a standard tablecloth – try using unusual fabrics such as sari material, a plaid rug, velvet or lace. Experiment and see how the fabric changes the mood and energy of the table. Make edible napkin holders out of rings of rosemary and chives – add sprigs of thyme, marjoram and parsley if you like. Instead of a central flower arrangement think of alternatives. Maybe scatter fresh herbs or petals over the table. Or give each person his or her own jam-jar of flowers. Individual tea-lights can look pretty too.

One nice little ritual is to visualize the whole table surrounded by a loving ball of vital energy.

Think about how you can make each person feel at home and comfortable. Seating plans may seem old-fashioned but they mean you can plan who sits where. The place at the top of the table is traditionally the place of honour – if you want to show respect place your grandparents or parents in this place. Difficult children can be kept in line by being placed next to such venerable figures! If you need to make a business person feel welcomed and comfortable, seat them opposite you so you can give them your undivided attention.

Use the old tradition of seating cards to make people feel especially welcome. At my wedding I put a hand-written note on the back of each card, with a message or memory of some past happy times. Equally you could put down an interesting fact about the person who is sitting next to your guest to instigate conversations. Of course, never forget that good seating plans have always been responsible for some wonderful romantic liaisons – energy at work in the best possible way!

Of course you don't have to eat at a table inside. Dining outdoors brings an elemental energy into mealtimes that is always slightly wild and unpredictable (and all the better for it). Take the opportunity to have picnics – in the woods, on the beach, up a mountain, in a city park, on a boat floating on a city boating lake! It doesn't have to be hot and it doesn't need to be daytime. Transform a garden or roof terrace into a magical outdoor room with loads of candles in jars or storm lanterns. Burn citronella to keep away the bugs. Wrap up warm and have a winter barbecue. Don't forget to sing songs and tell tales after the meal.

Bring back the old art of blessings and grace at mealtime. You don't have to use formal religious graces and you don't need to sit for hours while your food gets cold! One nice way of 'doing' grace is to have a moment's silent thanks before you start to eat. Or you could leave it until afterwards and then each say a word of thanks – to the food itself, to the gods, to the cook. Grace is a way of making us conscious of the food we eat and the way it came to our table.

Try to make your mealtimes warm, loving, peaceful occasions. One nice ritual is to visualize the whole table surrounded by a loving ball of vital energy. Imagine there is a cord reaching from the heart chakra of each person at the table – they all reach into the centre of the table where they meet and entwine. So everyone is linked to everyone else, in a swirling network of light and energy. This is particularly useful if you have a difficult meal in front of you.

Try to ensure that everyone has a say. When there are children, often the more confident will hog the conversation (not just children either!) Try to bring everyone into the conversation – not by putting them on the spot but by gently bringing the conversation round to a topic about which they are knowledgeable.

Feng shui, the Chinese art of placement, is all to do with energy. So naturally it has guidelines for good energy eating! The table should ideally be rounded and wooden. If this isn't possible, don't worry – but do make sure you represent all the elements on your table (a decanter of water or wine represents water; the cutlery represents metal; candles are for fire; flowers or herbs represent wood; china, glass and any stones or rocks you use as ornaments represent earth. Burn some essential oils or some subtle incense to include the air element.
Finally, keep the doors in your dining room shut while you are eating – otherwise the flow of energy might make you feel anxious and hurried.

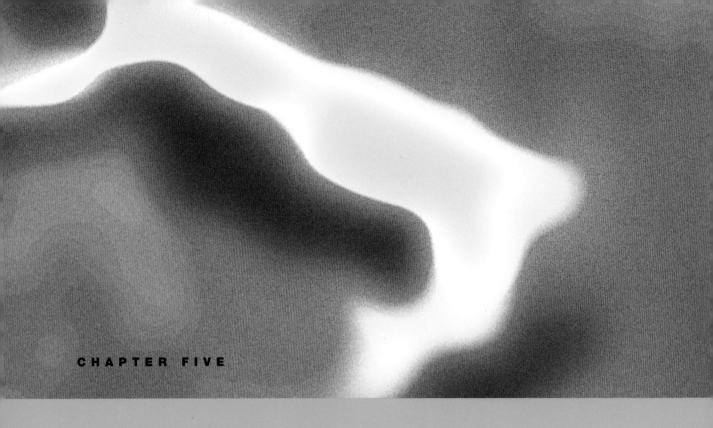

CHAPTER FIVE

ENERGY EXERCISE

If you really want to cultivate more energy in your body, in your life, then exercise. 'Oh but I haven't got the energy to exercise,' is a common complaint. Ironic, isn't it? Yet, however tired you may feel you are, the strange thing is that, if you start to exercise, you will very swiftly feel much better – healthier, happier, more energetic. This chapter is a bit like the one on food – you may feel a huge resistance to even reading about exercise, let alone doing it. Yet bear with me. The good news is that energy exercise is probably exactly the opposite to how you think of exercise. It does not preach 'no pain, no gain' – in fact far from it. You don't have to be up at the crack of dawn doing circuits round the park (unless, of course, that is your preferred form of exercise). In fact, plenty of exercises in this chapter involve little more than standing in one spot. Not too arduous?

We are all familiar with the notion that regular exercise is 'good' for the body – it keeps our hearts and lungs in good condition, stretches and tones the muscles and internal organs; it increases flexibility and staves off osteoporosis.

But first and foremost, why exercise at all? We are all familiar with the notion that regular exercise is 'good' for the body – it keeps our hearts and lungs in good condition, stretches and tones the muscles and internal organs; it increases flexibility and staves off osteoporosis. Exercising also releases endorphins, the 'feelgood' chemicals which enhance mood. It's even been said that regular exercise can promote a good sex life! But, as if all that were not enough, exercise is one of the prime ways of cultivating and balancing vital energy within the body. Good exercise can literally 'charge' the body, increasing the amount of healing vital energy within it.

So what constitutes 'good' exercise? Any exercise which is performed with grace and enjoyment can be healing. Many of us were put off 'sport' when we were at school because we just weren't good at the sports on offer. How many of us were humiliated on the running track, or dredged up excuse after excuse so as not to be put through the shame of failing yet again at gym? Me for one! I loathed sport at school because I simply wasn't the gymnastic type. 'Type' – now there's the clue – we are all different and just because you don't like one form of exercise doesn't mean you are not the exercise 'type'. No, you just have to find the form of exercise that suits you.

John Douillard, former athlete, coach and author of *Body, Mind and Sport* believes that we are all trying to force round pegs into square holes. He has applied ayurvedic principles to sport and exercise – with remarkable results. Children who formally hated sport, now love it. Athletes who were damaging both body and mind in search of perfection are now just as good, if not better, without the strain. So how does his bodymind sport work? Well, first you work out your bodymind type, known in Ayurveda as your prakruti. Then, if you are starting out, you simply choose a form of exercise that suits your prakruti. It's that simple but it works because you are working with, rather than against, your own internal energy.

Kapha people are usually heavier framed than vata or pitta. If you're a natural kapha you will have a strong body and great levels of endurance.

In practice, this is how it works. First, simply decide which of the three doshas, or bodymind energies, is most like you (most of us are combinations of two doshas but just pick the most similar).

Vata: If you have a lot of vata in your constitution, you will tend to be slim with an active mind and a restless body. You talk a lot, very fast, and ask lots of questions. In fact everything about you is fast – you walk fast, eat fast, sleep lightly. You learn quickly (but forget quickly too), you can't sit still for more than a moment. You have a vivid imagination and are highly creative and sensitive.

NATURAL INCLINATIONS IN EXERCISE: You are a natural sprinter or runner. You may be good at gymnastics. Pretty well any kind of field sport (with the exception of the shot put!) will suit you. Pick sports or exercise which capitalize on your speed and agility. If you play team sports put yourself in a position where the emphasis is on speed.

Pitta: Pitta people are usually in the middle – medium build, medium appetite, sleep for a middling amount of time, walk and talk with a medium speed. If you're a pitta you are a natural leader, strong-minded, fiery and quick-tempered. You have good coordination and can be very (VERY) competitive.

NATURAL INCLINATIONS IN EXERCISE: Pittas love competition and thrive under a bit of stress. So don't bore yourself rigid by taking up long distance running: join a team or get involved with a league. If that isn't possible then try to exercise with someone – competitive pitta will even get a kick out of meditating better than someone else!

Kapha: Kapha people are usually heavier framed than vata or pitta. If you're a natural kapha you will have a strong body and great levels of endurance. You tend to take life slower than your energetic counterparts – you walk steadily, eat slowly (but with a good appetite), learn slowly (but once you've learned it, it's there forever). You're a patient, generally kind-natured person.

NATURAL INCLINATIONS IN EXERCISE: Kaphas are built for endurance and strength so pick out sports needing these qualities. Any shot-putter is bound to be a kapha. You will also do well with team sports because you will thrive under the motivation of others. Anything involving distance works well too: whether long-distance swimming, cross-country running, race walking...

KEY CONCEPTS FOR ENERGY EXERCISING

To get the most out of any exercise there are two key concepts. The first should come as no surprise – it's breathing. John Douillard teaches every student of his to breathe through the nose at all times. This may seem strange if you are used to panting your way through an aerobics class or gasping for air, mouth wide open, as you run. But, he insists, this is the only way to harness healing energy and to allow the body to enjoy the benefits of exercise without over-stretching or stressing it. His 'Darth Vadar' breath is nothing more or less than the ujjayi form of yogic breathing, making a rasping sound with the out breath. To recap, do it this way:

● Breathe in through the nose.

● Breathe out through the nose, slightly constricting the throat so you make a guttural sound. You will feel a sensation in your throat, rather than in your nose.

● Notice that your stomach muscles slightly contract as you breathe out.

You will find at first that, breathing in this way, you can work for far less time. Don't panic. Just slow down your workout to suit your breath, your body. You will quickly find that, breathing in this way, you will be able to return to your former fitness levels – and even surpass them.

The second concept is mindfulness. By bringing awareness to your workout, you can become aware of the energy moving within the body. 'Even if you do just one minute, one full stretch, but with total intent, I believe it can rejuvenate you,' says Lydia Wong, who teaches her own form of exercise based on chi kung, tai chi and yoga.

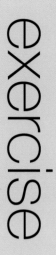

EXERCISE AS MEDITATION

You can also use exercise as a form of meditation. The easiest way to do this is with walking.

● As you walk, become aware of your feet on the ground. At first you can say to yourself, 'right foot, left foot,' as you feel each foot touch the ground.

● How does the ground feel? Make yourself as light as possible, so you literally tread lightly on the earth.

● Notice your breathing – make it as calm as possible (using the nasal breathing as above).

● How does your body feel? Become aware of any tension you may be holding.

● Are your thoughts intrusive? What is worrying you? Agree to lay it aside for the duration of your walk.

● Once you have become aware of your body as it walks, you can turn to the world around you. Notice the weather and how the hot/cold/damp/mist feels on your skin. Start to notice small things around you – the texture of the road, the cracks in the road, any flowers or weeds pushing through, for example. This is also a lovely way to tune yourself into the energy of the natural world – something we'll do far more of in Part Three.

SUPER ENERGY – ANCIENT EXERCISES TAILOR-MADE FOR TODAY

In fact, you don't even need to work out your ideal exercise – if you don't feel so inclined. There are some wonderful short-cuts – forms of exercise that automatically work with your internal energy to produce incredibly effective results. Once again we're turning to India and China where exercise has evolved, over thousands upon thousands of years, into a pure healing art, intended to cultivate and balance vital energy.

Yoga (from India) and chi kung (sometimes called qi gong) and tai chi (taiji) from China are pure energy exercise. More than that, they are profound healing methods. Just as Chinese physicians liked to use food before more aggressive healing methods, they would also prescribe chi kung which, with its combination of breathing, posture and meditation, could influence every part of the body, from the inside out. The very name chi kung translates as 'working with life energy' and it is a profound science which can pinpoint energy imbalances and correct them.

Chi kung is ideal exercise because absolutely anyone can do it. Even if you cannot stand up, you can perform the exercises sitting down! And while it may look effortless when performed by a master, in practise it is a precise discipline, demanding meticulous concentration and patience. It is also surprisingly tough on the muscles. I lift weights regularly but within a few minutes of chi kung my muscles were aching to a degree I normally experience only after a good 40 minutes in the gym.

Ideally you should practice chi kung every day, even if it is only for five or ten minutes. Obviously, though, the more effort you put in, the more results you will see. It's not a quick fix, but the more you practice it, the more it creates energy. This is perhaps the strangest aspect of chi kung – while other forms of exercise take away your energy, chi kung puts it back. And, while you won't burn calories, you will find your body shape changing as you practice the exercises as a result of the combined effects of the breathing, the movement and the liberation of chi.

Let's try a few very simple chi kung exercises to get the chi moving. If you find these enjoyable, it would be worth finding a good teacher in your area and pursuing it further.

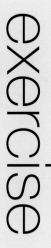

THE STARTING POSTURE

This is the basic posture of chi kung. It puts you in the correct position and helps you become aware of your entire body. If it seems familiar it's because we started this book with a modified version of it!

1. Stand with your feet shoulder-width apart. Find your natural balance – your weight should neither be too far forward nor too far back or it will cause tension and tiredness.

2. Feel the rim of your foot, your heel, your little toe and big toe relaxed on the ground.

3. Keep your knees relaxed. Check your knees are exactly over your feet.

4. Relax your lower back. Relax your stomach and buttocks.

5. Let your chest become hollow. Relax and slightly round your shoulders.

6. Imagine you have a pigtail on top of your head that is tied to a rafter on the roof. Let your head float lightly and freely. Relax your tongue, mouth and jaw.

7. Stay in this position for a few moments with your hands hanging loosely by your sides.

8. Take your mind through the five elements. Earth (imagine the feeling of weight and rootedness); Water (looseness and fluidity); Air (lightness and transparency); Fire (sparkle – remember this should be fun!); and Space (envisage the space within each joint, muscle, breath and mind).

9. Throughout your chi kung practice, keep bringing your mind gently back to your posture – this keeps the mind restful.

HOLDING THE DANTIEN

This exercise stimulates the dantien, which in chi kung is considered to be the storehouse of chi. It also helps circulation and lymph drainage and helps to promote deep, effective breathing. The dantien is located about an inch or so below the navel.

1. Stand in the Starting Posture.

2. Men should place their left hand on the dantien, and the right hand over the left. Women should place their right hand on the dantien with the left over it. Relax your whole body and concentrate your thoughts on the dantien.

3. With the legs straight but not locked, breathe into the dantien. You will feel your abdomen inflate under your hands.

4. Slowly bend your knees and breathe out. Your abdomen will deflate into the body on the out breath. Repeat this exercise for at least two minutes – as you get used to it, you can continue it for longer.

exercise

SUPPORTING THE SKY

This exercise is excellent for improving the energy exchange within the lungs and for balancing your breathing.

1. Stand in the Starting Posture.

2. Hold your hands in front of your dantien so the palms face up and the fingers point to each other.

3. Raise your hands up past the front of your chest so that the palms face the body. Breathe in. As your hands come up, keep your back straight and when the hands reach the face roll your hands over (so the palms face upwards). Stretch your arms up and look upwards.

4. Open your arms out to the sides and lower them down while bending the knees. Keep the back straight until the hands are in the Starting Posture but now with your knees bent. Breathe out at the same time. Repeat at least five or six times for the best benefit.

TURNING THE HEAD AND TWISTING THE TAIL

This exercise helps to improve kidney energy. It strengthens the spine and helps keep it flexible and strong. It takes a fair bit of coordination but do persist as it is highly effective.

1. Stand in the Starting Posture with the arms raised at the side of the body to shoulder height.

2. Place your weight in the right leg, keeping both legs bent. Lean to the left while raising your right arm slightly. Allow the left arm to curve downwards so the tips of your fingers touch your left thigh about where a trouser seam would be. Turn your head to look into the palm of the right hand. As you perform this move, exhale.

3. Come back to the starting position with your arms raised to the side of your body, breathing in as you return.

4. Now shift the weight into the left leg and lean to the right, raising your left arm slightly and curving the right arm downwards so the finger tips touch the right thigh. Turn your head to look into the palm of the right hand. Breathe out as you perform this move.

5. Repeat at least five times each side, keeping your movements slow and flowing.

DRAGON STAMPING

This exercise works wonders for your circulation and balance, both mental and physical. It helps to calm the mind and, if performed every morning, helps you become focused and energized for the day ahead. Make sure you are breathing out as you rise and in as you return – it's very easy to get it the wrong way round which is far less effective.

1. Stand in the Starting Posture.

2. Breathing out, go slowly right up onto your tiptoes, as high as you can. Stretch your body upwards through the back keeping the abdomen relaxed. At the same time point your fingers down and inwards, stretching your arms downwards.

3. Return your heels slowly to the ground on the in breath and relax. Repeat at least five times.

YOGA – MOBILIZING ENERGY

Yoga is becoming amazingly popular. It's not surprising as it really is a super-exercise, reaching parts other exercise systems haven't even thought of! Yoga postures put pressure on different organs very systematically. It tones the whole inner body as well as the outer body.

Yoga teachers claim that the precise asanas (postures) of yoga work deep into the body, causing blood to circulate deeply, nourishing every organ and softening the muscle and ligament tissue. The deep stretching is said to bring both bones and muscles gently back into their optimum alignment while lubricating the joints. Best of all, yoga is superlatively good at mobilizing vital energy. You emerge from a session feeling that weird combination of relaxed yet energized because yogic breathing directly affects the nervous system. John Douillard raves about yoga. He found that by using yoga postures (in particular a series known as the sun salute) and breathing practice he could help people achieve maximum fitness – without the pain of hard aerobic training.

If you have been following this book from the beginning you have already practised yoga! The breathing exercises in Chapter One come mainly from pranayama, the science of yogic breathing. Once you have mastered the breath, the asanas will often come quite easily. I recommend you find a good teacher if you want to explore yoga properly. The asanas are very precise and no video can really fine-tune your poses. However, because this is primarily a practical book, I'm going to run through a series of exercises that is an ideal introduction to yoga.

exercise

Doing yoga is like giving yourself

an energy shower

exercise

THE SUN SALUTE – A COMPLETE WORKOUT FOR BODY, MIND AND SPIRIT
In ancient India the sun salute was part of daily spiritual practice and was performed in the very early morning facing the sun. Why not start your day this way and tap into the universal energy of the sun?

Start off with just one whole set and gradually build up to the optimum 12. You may find it helpful to record the instructions on tape until you become familiar with them.

POSTURE ONE: Standing upright, bring your feet together so your big toes are touching. Your arms are by your sides. Relax your shoulders and tuck your chin in slightly – look straight ahead, not down at your feet. Bring your hands together in front of your chest with palms together as if you were praying. Exhale deeply.

POSTURE TWO: Inhale slowly and deeply while you bring your arms straight up over your head, placing your palms together as you finish inhaling. Softly look backwards towards your thumbs. Lift the knees by tightening your thighs. Reach up as far as possible, lengthening your whole body. If you feel comfortable you can take the posture back slightly further into a bend.

POSTURE THREE: Exhale as you bend forwards so that your hands are in line with your feet. Your head should be touching your knees. To begin with you might find you have to bend your knees in order to reach. Eventually you should be able to straighten your knees into the full posture.

POSTURE FOUR: Inhale deeply and move your left leg away from your body in a big backwards sweep so you end up in a kind of extended lunge position. Keep your hands and right foot firmly on the ground. Your right knee should be between your hands. Bend your head upwards, stretching out your back.

POSTURE FIVE: Exhaling deeply, bring your right leg back and push your hips up into an inverted 'v' posture. Your arms are in front of your head, palms facing directly in front, arms shoulder-width apart. Your back should be in a straight line with your head in line with your arms. Keep your feet and heels flat on the floor.

POSTURE SIX: Exhale and lower your body onto the floor. Only eight parts of your body should be in contact with the floor: your feet, your knees, your hands, your chest and your forehead. Try to keep your abdomen raised and, if you can possibly manage it, keep your nose off the floor so only your forehead makes contact. Don't worry if it's an impossibility at this point – just keep the idea in mind.

POSTURE SEVEN: Inhale and bend up into the position known as the cobra. Hands on the floor in front of you, arms straight and bend backwards as far as feels comfortable. Look upwards.

POSTURE EIGHT: Exhale and lift your back back into posture five (known as the dog). Remember to keep your feet and heels (if you can) flat on the floor.

POSTURE NINE: Inhale and return to posture four, this time with the opposite leg forwards. So your left foot is in line with your hands while your right leg is stretched back.

POSTURE TEN: Exhale and return to posture three.

POSTURE ELEVEN: Raise the arms overhead and bend backwards as you inhale (as for posture two).

POSTURE TWELVE: Return to a comfortable standing position, feet together, arms by your sides. Look straight ahead and exhale. To close, bring your hands back together in a position of prayer.

exercise

exercise

Further yoga postures for health and vitality

As you become more proficient in yoga, you can extend your practice. Once you have performed your sun salutations, you may like to include these postures, all of which will help to increase vital energy. Perform them slowly and carefully in a controlled manner. Never race.

THE MOUNTAIN

This seated variation of the mountain posture tones your abdominal muscles and improves your breathing. It can help sluggish circulation and can also tone the muscles in the back.

1. Sit cross-legged on the floor. Hold yourself upright and breathe naturally and easily.

2. Inhale and stretch your arms up over your head to form a steeple shape over your head. Keep the insides of your arms close to your ears. Bring your palms together if you can and press them together as if you were praying. Imagine you are a mountain, solid, powerful and strong. Bring this wonderful mountain energy into your body and into your life.

3. Hold this posture for as long as you can, comfortably. Remember to breathe easily and regularly as you hold the pose.

4. Exhale and slowly lower your arms to your lap. Rest for a few moments and then repeat.

PRAYER POSTURE

This gentle posture puts all your internal organs into balance. It encourages deep breathing and helps to align your spine into its optimum position. It is also deeply calming for the mind.

1. Stand with your feet together and parallel. Aim to stand tall without straining – imagine you have a string fastening your head to the ceiling.

2. Check your head – it should be easily balanced on your neck with eyes gazing softly ahead. Your chin should be neither tucked in or jutting out.

3. Tilt your pelvis slightly forwards and keep your knees straight but soft – don't lock them.

4. Now bring your hands together in front of your chest, as if you were praying.

5. Relax your jaw, your facial muscles and your shoulders. Breathe softly and regularly. You may want to focus lightly on an object in front of you – or you can gently close your eyes.

6. Hold this pose for a few minutes or as long as you feel comfortable. Then bring your hands back down to your sides and resume your normal stance.

THE TREE
A classic yoga posture which is superb for improving your balance, concentration and coordination.

1. Stand up tall and straight. Your feet should be close together and parallel. Fix your eyes gently on a spot ahead and breathe naturally and regularly. You will need to keep your eyes open for this posture.

2. Lift one leg and place the sole of your foot against the inner side of your other thigh. You can use your hands to help. (Note – if this is impossible, don't worry – bring your foot up as high as you can: it might only be to your ankle at first.) Keep focusing on the point ahead of you.

3. Now bring your hands up in a prayer position in front of your chest.

4. Hold the posture for as long as feels comfortable. Focus on your breathing and think about the strength and poise of a tree – its roots firm in the ground; its branches reaching towards heaven. Think about its flexibility too – how it bends in the wind. Bring this energy into your body and into your life – it will be very useful in our stressful society.

5. Repeat the posture on the other side.

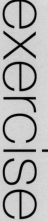

THE ENERGY OF THE DANCE

Don't panic if you've reached this far in the chapter and still don't feel like exercising! I have one last hope of catching you. Often people don't like the idea of yoga and chi kung because they seem too static and boring. Actually they aren't, but I can understand the point. Most of us are caught up in the very yang energy of our frenetic society – we can't relate to something soft and quiet. So, if you crave something more primally energetic, try dance.

Not just any dance though. Certain forms of dance have the ability to plug straight into vital energy. In fact, in many ancient cultures, dance was considered a way to the gods, a form of healing. For example, the Kung San of the Kalahari Desert, use dance to activate 'num', their term for vital energy. Num, they believe, is stored in the lower abdomen and at the base of the spine. By dancing, you can make the num 'boil' and can, if trained, project the healing energy to other people or pull out sick energy from those who are unwell.

However you don't need to go to the Kalahari desert to find healing energy through the dance. There are several forms of healing dance available in the West, including Biodanza.

Biodanza

Biodanza was created by Chilean psychologist and anthropologist Rolando Toro in 1960. He recognized that tribal societies have always used dance as a way to express deep feelings and to connect both to one another and to society as a whole. It was an energy exchange. Toro felt that we can literally dance ourselves back to wholeness. Working initially with mentally disturbed patients, he found that certain kinds of music would evoke certain kinds of movements, which would, in turn, bring about quite pronounced physiological and emotional changes.

He came to believe that each of us has within us five different energetic modes of living: Vitality (feeling energy, facing the world); Affectivity (feelings of love, tenderness and respect; giving and receiving from others); Sexuality (deriving pleasure from our sensual energy); Creativity (bringing creative energy into everyday life) and Transcendence (going beyond ego to find something powerful outside ourselves). Our problems arise because we learn to stifle some or all of these living experiences and so fall out of our natural balance. The idea behind Biodanza is to try to bring the whole person back into a childlike sense of wholeness by stimulating underdeveloped areas and bringing all five into balance.

HOME DANCE CLASS

In Biodanza every exercise and its accompanying music is carefully planned to have a precise physiological effect. However, you can try the following exercises to experience a taste of Biodanza in your own home.

1. Walk around the room, or garden, and try to feel connected with your body. Feel your feet connecting firmly with the ground; let your arms swing naturally and keep your head up high. Gradually let the movement become more fluid, more vital, more exuberant.

2. Put on music with a strong but fluid melody. Dance in any way you choose, but remain aware of your chest and heart area and dance 'into' that area.

3. Change the music for something with a solid, firm rhythm. Dance again, but this time letting your movements be governed by your pelvic region.

4. Keep with rhythmic music and play with finding your 'own' dance. Forget notions of what dancing should look like; don't worry about proper steps or movements. Allow the music to dance you – you might end up jumping in the air, or rolling on the floor: it doesn't matter.

5. Again, pick some music with a firm beat and practise giving your dance to someone else. If you are trying these exercises with a friend, one of you should sit on the floor and 'receive' the dance while you dance for her/him. If you are doing this alone, imagine you are dancing for someone special and pretend they are sitting in front of you. Again, let the music guide you in your movements and concentrate on really giving the other person what they need. Maintain eye contact all the way through the exercise. Then swap over and receive their dance.

There's absolutely no need to be a 'good' dancer. Unlike yoga and chi kung, there is no 'correct' way of doing this form of dance, the whole point is to find your own dance.

exercise

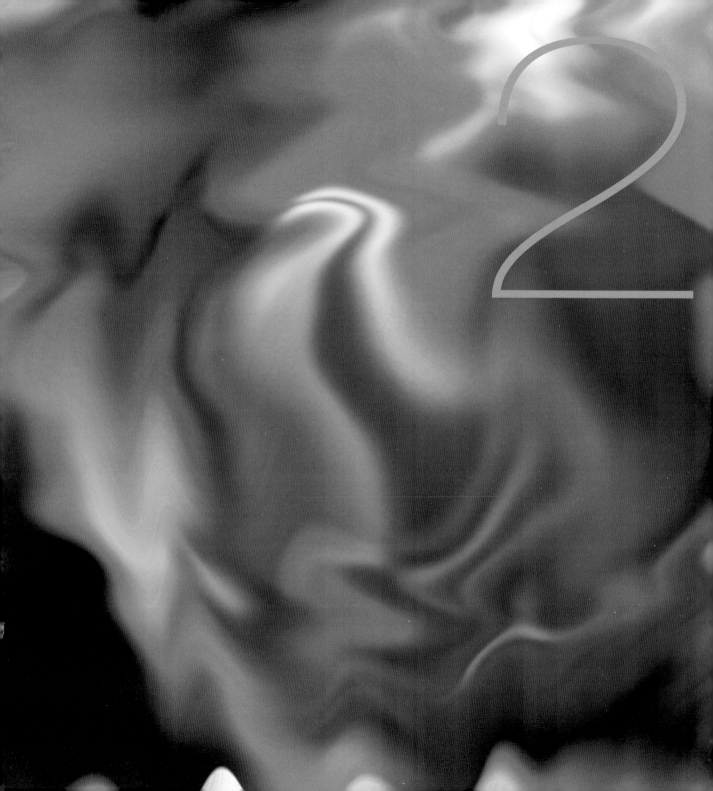

2

emotional**energy**

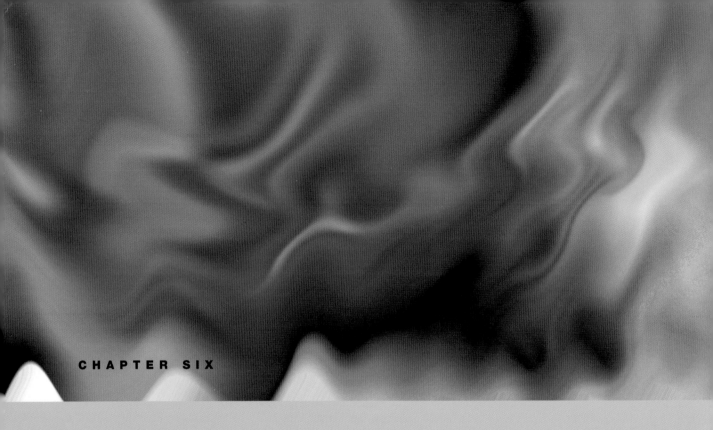

CHAPTER SIX

WORKING WITH EMOTIONAL ENERGY

Energy is not just a physical thing – far from it. While we can feel energy moving it our bodies, we can also detect it at work in our emotions, our minds, our interactions with other people. Think about it. You wake up and it's Monday morning, you have a meeting you are dreading with a person you hate. So how do you feel? Now imagine you wake up and it's Saturday morning: ahead of you lies a day at the beach with your family or a group of great friends. Does that feel different? You bet it does! Learning how to shift your emotional energy can be a huge boon in modern life. It won't take the traumas and unpleasantness out of everyday life but it will enable you to deal with it in the best possible way.

Many therapists now think that our emotional energy can become blocked, warped or repressed at a very early age. Some go as far as suggesting that even our time in the womb can be formative.

Emotional energy manifests itself in our moods, our feelings and attitudes. If you have vital energy freely moving through you, you will tend to have a sunny disposition, an optimistic outlook, a frank, open and honest approach to the world. If your energy is blocked you will probably show some of the classic symptoms which we tend to think of as vices or psychological problems: for example anger, fear, jealousy, resentment, shame.
But what causes this blockage in the first place? Many therapists now think that our emotional energy can become blocked, warped or repressed at a very early age. Some go as far as suggesting that even our time in the womb can be formative.

Take a few moments to consider the following questions. You may like to sit down quietly when you know you won't be disturbed. Perhaps light a candle to focus your mind.

● If your parents are alive, ask them about your earliest beginnings. Were you planned or a 'surprise'? How were you conceived? What emotions surrounded the news of your existence? If your parents are no longer alive, is there anyone else you can ask? Siblings, aunts, uncles, your parents' friends?

● How was your mother's pregnancy? Did she have any physical problems? How were her emotions? Was there any stress? Any financial worries?

● What kind of birth did you have? Were you early, on time or late? Did your mother have to have any drugs, any surgical intervention? Was she frightened? Was the birth easy or difficult, short or very long?

● How was your babyhood and early childhood? What is your earliest memory?

● What do you remember most about your childhood? What emotions did you express most freely? Which emotions were you not allowed, or not encouraged to express? For example, were you told off for being too loud or too boisterous?

● Did you suffer any traumas as a child? Did you lose a parent or watch your parents divorce? Was there illness in the family, or poverty, or severe stress?

It's worth making the effort to dig out this information. You might find out some surprising facts. As babies and children we are incredibly open to suggestion – we are like little psychic sponges. The actions, words and emotions of the people who surround us will literally make up how we experience the world. And how we experience the world, our world view, will affect our own emotional energy. If we were over-protected as children, not allowed to run free, the world can appear a dangerous place – our own emotional energy shrinks back in fear. If we were not given enough warmth and cuddling, the world can appear cold and unwelcoming – our energy surrounds us in a cocoon to keep us warm (but keeps out other people). If we were hurt, ignored, pushed aside, our energy will try to protect us by building a wall around our feelings – which, of course, keeps out the good as well as the bad.

Parents have the trickiest of jobs – it's a perilously difficult dance to give a child the emotional grounding he or she needs: sensing that there are times to be warm and enclosing, protective in your love and at other times allowing the child the freedom and space to go out and explore, to push back the frontiers. Of course you won't get it right all the time – and of course our own parents didn't. It's important to say that this exercise of looking back should never become a source of recrimination. What's done is done and cannot be changed – except by taking charge of your own energy here and now, in the present. It's useful to know the earliest roots of your emotional blockages but it's fruitless to waste time in blame.

exercise

TRACKING UNWANTED EMOTIONAL ENERGY

Another way of uncovering the underlying negative emotions that are stifling our energy flow is to work with your body. Choose a time when you won't be disturbed, ideally somewhere where you can make a noise if you want. You might choose to have some cushions or pillows around you. Note: if you feel overly anxious about doing this exercise, you might want to have someone you totally trust with you. If it feels very scary, maybe you need to explore this area with some professional help.

● Lie down on the floor, on a comfortable mat or rug.

● Spend some time centring yourself, breathing slowly and deeply.

● Become aware of your body. Where are you holding tension? Where do you feel discomfort? Pinpoint the place and the feeling.

● Now exaggerate the feeling. So, if you are clenching your jaw, clench it harder. And harder.

● What does your body want to do or say? Don't think, just let your body follow its need. You might find yourself spitting out words or phrases; you might curl up in a ball; you might lash out at a cushion...you might do nothing.

● Give your body permission to do whatever it needs to express its repressed emotional energy – within safe limits.

● When you feel your body has had enough for this session, lie quietly once more and return to your breathing.

● Stand up and stamp your feet to return to normal awareness. You may wish to write down what happened.

The issues may not be clear the first time you try this. It may be worth re-reading the section on chakras, as where we hold tension is often directly related to our emotional blockages. As a brief guideline:

● the eye area tends to be about what we are allowed to see

● the mouth/jaw/throat area tends to be about communication, about being heard, about nourishment

● the chest and heart area tends to be about anger, sadness, rejection, longing

● the abdominal area tends to be about fear and digestion (what we take in)

● the pelvic/sacral area tends to be about sexuality, survival, support, vitality.

Our bodies really do know the answers. Bodyworkers have found that repressed thoughts, feelings, hurts and memories are all stored in the body. If you feel you have a lot of old psychological 'baggage' but are nervous of trying psychotherapy, I recommend you go to a good bodyworker. Many people find that, under the skilled hands of a therapist, they can release old patterns, allowing their emotional energy to run free once more. Sometimes you recall the old hurts – sometimes you don't have to relive the experience, just let it go.

Keep a journal – record your dreams

While you are doing this work it really is worthwhile keeping a log of your experiences and feelings. Use it for writing down what you discover during the exercises in this book. Use it to record your dreams, stray thoughts, meditations and visualizations.

I would also heartily recommend you start recording your dreams. Dreams offer incredible pointers to our energetic state. But it can take some time to figure out their language. Dreams speak in riddles, in symbols and images rather than straightforward messages. So write down your dream and then spend some time thinking about it, however silly it might appear.

● If some particular object or animal appears in your dream think about what it means to you. What significance does that thing have for you? What does it remind you of? Allow your mind to work laterally.

● Other people who appear in dreams are often aspects of ourselves – perhaps those that are repressed or not allowed to express themselves freely. Animals can represent our 'animal' side too. A great technique for understanding this form of energy is to hold a 'conversation' with a character or animal in a dream. Imagine it is sitting opposite you (behind a solid glass wall, if it's scary) – ask it what it wants, what it needs. You might just be surprised.

● Another technique for working with dreams is to 'dream the dream on'. Lie or sit down and breathe deeply so you become calm and centred. Imagine yourself back in your dream. Run through the dream as you remember it but, instead of it ending, allow it to continue. Imagine what would happen next. You can also choose this way of conversing with figures and animals.

● Painting is a wonderful way of moving dream work too. You don't need to be an artist – far from it. Simply put out a large piece of paper and use whatever materials you desire. You can either draw your dream figuratively or just let the paint express how you felt in the dream. Whichever, don't censor yourself – just let the paint talk. After you have finished, sit back and look. What can you see? Does anything become clearer? Did any emotions come up as you were painting? Maybe write to your painting – or dance the feelings it brings up in you.

These are all very powerful techniques and we're rushing through them at a rate of knots! So please don't feel you have to do everything at once. Take it slowly, in your own time and at your own pace. Many of us spent our childhoods being told to either 'hurry up' or 'slow down' – time is one of the dimensions into which our energy was moulded from a very tender age. So give yourself the time you need. Do remember also that these are the kind of techniques that are often used in a therapeutic setting – with trained therapists on hand. I tend to follow the great spiritual workshop leader Denise Linn's belief that we will go no further than we are ready to – that our psyches have a way of protecting us from going too far, too quickly. So, if you feel happy about these exercises, then you should be perfectly OK to do them. If you feel the slightest doubt, proceed with caution or not at all.

LIBERATING EMOTIONAL ENERGY

By now hopefully you have some idea of where your emotional energy blockages are and how they got there. Now you have to shift them. First and foremost, remember that these blocks are there for good reason. Your energy hasn't done this for no reason – it is trying to protect you. So, before all else, thank the energy for being so protective and clever in thinking up ways of holding back painful memories and old hurts. Then ask it if it is willing to leave. Tell it that you are ready to move on, to become more open, more vulnerable, yes – more unprotected. You may find you feel a sense of something lifting, shifting, moving away from you. Bless it and imagine it dispersed in a flash of pure white shimmering light, transmuted into something pure, able to return to the source.

Of course, energy that has been lodged, often for years, may not be so easy to shift. Like a stubborn stain, it might take weeks, months, even years to resolve. Don't be in a hurry over this. Let it evolve naturally. Already, in this book, you have a host of tools to help dissolve old stuck energy (a choice of energy 'cleansers'). Work with the following:

● Breathe. Try practising the breathing exercises on a regular basis. If you have an area that feels stuck, try breathing into it, visualizing healing energy clearing away the blocks.

● Dance. Allowing your body to move as it wants can be hugely effective. Start with the biodanza moves on page 77 and then just let your body move in the way it wants. Or persist with the energy awareness exercise earlier in this chapter, exaggerating movements.

● Paint. Continue painting in a completely free fashion. If you find this hard, you could try painting with your non-dominant hand (i.e. if you're left-handed, paint with your right, and vice versa). Or paint with your eyes shut. Or paint to music. Or use clay.

● Dream. Continue with a dream diary and work with the images and symbols you discover.

● Find a good bodyworker or psychotherapist. My ideal is someone trained in both therapeutic talking and touching – biodynamic therapy and SHEN merge this well and many bodyworkers are now training in counselling too.

● Affirm. Choose an affirmation that digs to the heart of your block, for example, 'I am totally loveable.' 'It's safe to express my feelings.' 'I can be as loud as I like.' Write it 20 times, adding responses. Do this every day for 28 days and you may well find a lot of stuck energy emerging. Some responses may be a word; some might consist of pages of thoughts or memories. To reinforce the message, try saying your affirmation to yourself in a mirror. Note: the best affirmations are the ones that initially make your skin crawl!

The first step to freeing up our emotional energy is

to know where the blockages are and how they got there

DEALING WITH OTHER PEOPLE'S ENERGY

Once we have an understanding of our own nature, we are immediately in a much stronger position. When we are functioning from our true nature, rather than from behind the walls, screens and other defences of repressed energy, we gain a wonderful clarity. Often we automatically find that our relationships – with friends, family, workmates, complete strangers – are much clearer, more honest, more straightforward. When we no longer have to keep up the energy of pretending to be someone we are not, we can use all our energy to enjoy being ourselves!

However, just because we have sorted out ourselves does not mean that everyone else will have sorted out their own stuck energy. So, until the world becomes full of enlightened energyworkers, we have to learn how to deal with other people's stuck stuff.

It can be very unpleasant. You know the kind of people I'm talking about. You feel your spirits dip when they walk up to you. You find you're exhausted after just a few moments talking to them. They seem like psychic vampires, sucking out all your energy, all your vitality. Or they are just plain unpleasant – nasty bullies, emotional blackmailers, manipulative, sly and downright horrible.

Before you do anything else, you should feel pity for them. You know just how unpleasant it feels to walk around loaded down with heavy, stuck energy. So how do you think they feel? In fact one of the strongest techniques you can use is also the most simple. It simply entails sending pure loving energy to the person causing you grief. Here's how:

● **Centre yourself and focus on your breathing. Note: you can do this anywhere without the person even knowing.**

● **Now direct your awareness to your heart chakra – feel the chakra spinning steadily.**

● **Imagine a pure golden-white stream of divine universal energy coming shooting through your crown chakra and down into your heart. The whole chakra becomes full to bursting with this wonderful, loving, pure energy.**

exercise

● Send it out to the difficult person. Imagine it hitting them in the heart chakra and infusing their body with love and light. Be careful not to play games with this. Just send the loving energy – don't try to be clever and send wishes (for example 'let them be nice,' or anything like that).

That's it. I used to use this on a very difficult boss I once had. She would come in like an avenging fury and the whole office would beg me to do something about her. I used to quietly sit and direct this energy at her, repeating, 'I love you. I love you. I love you.' Which was very hard work! But it did work. She could tell something was happening as well because she would look suspicious and say 'What are you doing to me?' But that's the great thing about energywork – you leave no clues!

Sheilding techniques

Whilst the technique above is very useful for people you know and have to deal with on a day-to-day basis (because, eventually, it just might nudge them into a new way of being), there are other methods that are more effective for dealing with strangers.

The classic protection technique is the energy bubble. I've come across this – or forms of it – in virtually every tradition under the sun. It's very simple, very effective and can be used anywhere. This is my version...

● Breathe into your solar plexus and feel that chakra strong and responsive, centring you. Breathe into your root chakra and feel that chakra powerful, rooting you to the Earth. Breathe into your third eye chakra, feeling that chakra respond with clear vision and foresight. The chakras link up so it feels as though a rod of pure light is holding up your backbone.

● Now pull in pure energy from the universe through the crown chakra. Bring it down to the solar plexus and, from there, let it burst out around you into a bubble of pure, brilliant light which totally surrounds your body like a balloon.

● Know that no negative energy can come in through this powerful protective bubble – you are completely safe.

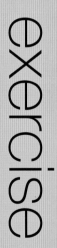

exercise

There are variations on this. I find the bubble the most effective for generally nerve-wracking situations or with people I find uncomfortable. If, however, you feel someone is deliberately targeting you with negative energy you might like to go one step further. Follow the first steps of the bubble technique – linking in with the chakras and pulling down the energy. But this time send it out into the shape of a large box – whose outward-facing sides are mirrors. This way, the negative energy that is thrown at you will bounce straight back to the person who sent it, which can be a very uncomfortable experience for them. Once you have 'disarmed' them this way, it could be the time to send that loving energy (if you are feeling particularly philanthropic).

Many of you may feel you have a particular guardian or guardians – angels, gods, goddesses, spirits, ancestors, animal allies. If so, by all means call on them for help in your energy-shielding exercises.

Guardians and allies

Despite the huge cynicism, agnosticism and atheism of this confused time, many people do have a strong sense of faith – if not for a particular religion, then for a deep-rooted spirituality. Many of you may feel you have a particular guardian or guardians – angels, gods, goddesses, spirits, ancestors, animal allies. If so, by all means call on them for help in your energy-shielding exercises. You could have the four archangels guarding your bubble – or infuse the bubble with the symbol for Ohm or an image of the Buddha. Or reverberate a holy name through the bubble.

I work a lot with the Native American power animals – simply because they resonate for me and seem to help me a lot. You could try this simple visualization to call on their energy. I use this whenever I need an energetic boost – when I have to go on a long journey, when I have to give a presentation or have a particularly important meeting. I find it very comforting and surprisingly energizing.

- Stand upright and breathe into your solar plexus.

- Feel your feet firmly on the ground, connecting with Mother Earth. Remember your roots, keep steady and true. You are a child of the Earth.

- Feel your head reaching up, connecting with Father Sky. Your feet may be rooted to the Earth but your aspirations reach to the sky, to the universe beyond. You are also a child of the Heavens.

- Now before you rises up the great animal spirit of Eagle. A huge powerful eagle turns and looks at you with his glimmering, all-seeing eye. You nod your head in acknowledgment and thanks. Eagle turns and spreads his wings. Now you will see through Eagle's eyes, enjoying his sharp far-sighted vision.

- Behind you rears up another huge figure – this time a great grizzly bear. You turn and look up into her sharp eyes, noticing her huge claws and her vast weight and strength. She is fiercely protective – who better to guard your back? Thank Bear and turn back, secure with her powerful presence behind you.

- You hear a sniff to your right, as if someone is trying to attract your attention. It's Coyote, his bright eyes dancing, his tongue lolling out as if he were laughing. Coyote is quick-talking, smart and a born negotiator. He can help you in any tricky situation. Be wary though – he's also a trickster. Don't let yourself become too clever for your own good or Coyote's strength becomes a weakness.

- Finally you feel a warm, sweet breath on your left arm. Turn and look into the dark melting eyes of Buffalo. She stands four-square, solid and dependable. Buffalo will help off-set tricky Coyote, keeping you grounded and stable.

- Spend a moment feeling these great guardians all around you. Now you can walk into any situation feeling protected and powerful. (Remember at the end of the meeting or day to thank your guardians – it's traditional to offer a prayer and a pinch of tobacco or cornmeal.)

exercise

CREATING ENERGETIC RAPPORT

Of course, we don't always need to keep people at arm's length. Sometimes we want to do exactly the opposite – to bring them closer. I wanted to discuss the shielding and protective techniques first because, sadly, there tends to be a lot of negative energy in the world and it's important to know how to close yourself off from it. But now it's time to talk about opening exercises, designed to create rapport and a kind of energy exchange. It is also vital preparatory work for our next chapter in which we look at love energy.

With what you already know about energy and how to move it around the body, you could probably work these techniques out for yourself! There is nothing mysterious about them and, if you can think of alternatives, try them out and see how they work. However, these ways are tried and trusted – and they work (at least for me)...

There are two basic bonding exercises. One for two of you working together and one where you are working without the other person knowing. If you possibly can, always try the former.

exercise

SOLO EXERCISE

● Centre yourself as always, breathing into your heart chakra this time.

● Bring down the loving energy from the crown chakra into the heart chakra and feel your heart fill with love and respect and caring for the other person.

● Spend a moment being quite clear about what you want to achieve. Remember you can't try to change them – just to open up the channels so you can have a more direct, honest communication. It's worth remembering that you can't make someone fall in love with you this way either!

● Send out a question to their heart chakra. Are they willing to receive your energy? Are they prepared to be open? Listen to your intuition.

● If the answer is yes, then gently send out a golden-pink stream of loving energy from your heart chakra to theirs. Imagine that, in return, they send the same back to you.

● Send a word of thanks to the universal source of all energy for allowing this exchange.

The very best energywork is that which we customize and invent for ourselves, using our own energetic pathways and thought processes

You can adapt these exercises depending on the situation. If, for example, you need to have an open discussion it might be more effective to exchange energy at the throat chakra – the energy here might be a pure clear blue. If you are going on a hard physical expedition you might exchange energy at the root level (for survival and stability), at the solar plexus (for courage and determination) and at the throat (for good communication).

JOINT EXERCISE

● Sit down or stand opposite each other. Centre yourselves as usual, breathing into your heart chakras.

● Bring down the energy through the crown chakra to the heart chakra and hold it there for a moment. At this point you can either say out loud what you want to achieve or just affirm it silently to yourselves.

● Now send the energy out into a bubble that surrounds the pair of you. Feel the two energies mixing and mingling, becoming stronger as a consequence. Realize with wonder that the two together become even stronger than the two apart.

● Now, if you wish, you can choose to link yourselves at the various chakras. This can be very powerful so, if you aren't totally sure of the person, I would recommend you leave it at the bubble stage. If you want to, however, link at whichever chakras seem appropriate.

● Be very respectful of each other's energy. Do not barge in – ask permission at each chakra.

exercise

COLOUR ENERGY

Sometimes it isn't as simple as 'good' people and 'bad' people. Sometimes you just don't know where a person is coming from; if their energy is positive or negative. And, to be fair, sometimes they don't know either. You will find, as your experience and confidence in energyworking grows that you usually have a fair idea. But if you're not sure then try this. Start visualizing the energy coming from everyone you meet as having a colour. If you have mastered reading auras, this will come in very useful now. But, if not, don't worry. When someone starts talking to you, let your intuition tell you what colour the energy they are directing towards you might be. If you don't know, imagine you do. What might it be? This may sound slightly strange but it's curiously effective. Someone might sound very nice and be smiling and appear warm but when you visualize their colour it could be an unpleasant dirty grey with flashes of dingy yellow or red. You might be uncovering their true feelings towards you – perhaps they feel jealous or uncertain or suspicious. Check back on the aura colour correspondences on pages 15 and 16.

If you feel threatened by this you can use a shielding technique, as we've already discussed. But, if you're feeling OK in yourself, you can try a far more beneficial exercise. Open your mouth slightly and breathe in the coloured energy. Take it down into your solar plexus area where your strong chakra energy whisks up the energy and transmutes it to a pure clear colour, say soft rose pink or gold. Then softly bring up this new energy and gently breathe it out towards the person. Keep practising this energy exchange until you detect a difference. Often you will find the person's attitude will change quite dramatically.

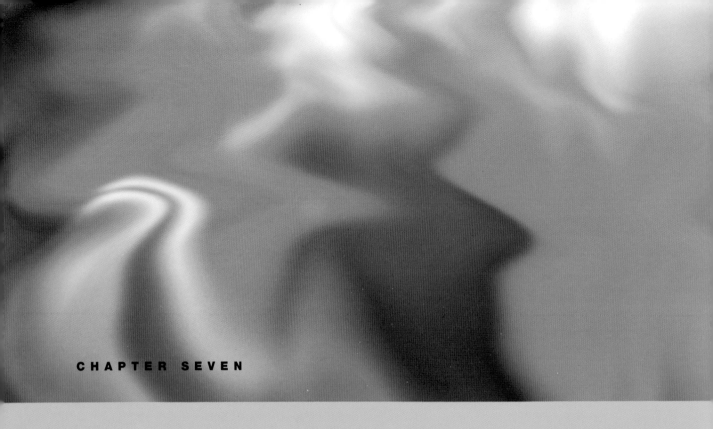

CHAPTER SEVEN

SEXUAL ENERGY

You probably think you know all there is to know about sex. After all, you can't buy a magazine nowadays without it telling you some new way to improve your sex life! If the number of books and videos on sex is anything to go by we should all be super-orgasmic. Yet most of this sex talk focuses on the pure mechanics of sexual activity. It just doesn't see sex for what it really is – an incredible energy exchange and force for both emotional and spiritual revitalization. Once again here in the West we have missed the boat. In the East the art of lovemaking has been a sacred energy art for many thousands of years. In India, Tibet and China (to name just a few) sex is taken very seriously indeed. It is approached with a deep sense of awe and respect – in many sects, such as Tantra, it is considered sacred, a form of divine worship. Tantra is a form of yoga, said to have been practised for over 6,000 years. It was originally one of many paths to spiritual, rather than sensual, enlightenment. While other forms of yoga employed physical training or meditation to reach unity with the Divine, Tantra used sexual union. In its purest form, Tantra turns sexuality into a meditation, almost a kind of worship. Tantra is technically a religion of sensuality – its church is the bedroom; its altar is your partner's body; its sacrament is sex.

Tantra teaches us to merge ecstatically with our partner and, through him or her, with the rest of the world.

The theory is that the universe was once blissfully united, whole. In Tantric mythology this was symbolized by the endless joyous intercourse of the female and male divinities, the goddess Shakti and the god Shiva. Then the universe split into two: Shakti and Shiva were separated and creation became divided into positive and negative energies, light and darkness, male and female. So now we suffer the pain of separation and it is this loneliness that apparently causes all the sorrow and suffering in the world. Subconsciously, we still remember a fragment of the bliss of union and constantly yearn to be back in that innocent state of primordial harmony. So the ultimate aim of Tantra is to reproduce that original divine union on a human scale. Tantra teaches us to merge ecstatically with our partner and, through him or her, with the rest of the world.

I first came across Tantra years ago and found it utterly fascinating. Although the full practice is intense and incredibly difficult, many of the exercises can be easily adapted for 'everyday' use and – although much watered-down – can have an incredible effect on your sex life!

Sexual energy is a highly potent force – some researchers believe the emerging sexuality of pubescent teenagers can cause poltergeist disturbance

BRINGING SACRED SEXUALITY INTO EVERYDAY LIFE

The first step in raising sexual energy is to accept that there is far more to sex than a quick thrill. You start by honouring your own body, accepting it as beautiful – whatever its size, shape or age.

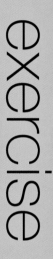

1. Choose a time when you will not be disturbed. You will need a full-length mirror and some candles; the room you use should be warm enough for you to feel comfortable without your clothes on.

2. Light the candles around the mirror and dim the lights. If you like you can light some incense (something gentle, loving and warm) or burn some aromatherapy oils (I would choose geranium, lavender, ylang-ylang or sandalwood).

3. Take off your clothes and sit in front of the mirror. Now look at your body. Resist the temptation to criticize. Instead of focusing on the bits you dislike, find a part you like. Your first thought might be that you dislike all of it ... but is that really true? Do you hate your fingers? Your wrists? Your ear-lobes? Your nostrils? Even if there is just one tiny bit that is OK, focus on that.

4. Think of the job it does – how wonderfully clever your fingers are, so dexterous and nimble; how miraculous your hearing is.

5. Just sit quietly with your body – for a good 20 minutes if you can.

When I first tried this, at the insistence of a Kahuna (a Hawaiian shaman and healer) I absolutely hated it. I loathed my body. Yet if you persist you may start to realize just how tough we are on our bodies. You may even start to like your body, to appreciate it. Truly we cannot expect to enjoy soaring sex and vibrant sensual energy, if we are battling against the flesh! So persist with this exercise – do it whenever you can. Always find something new that you like. Before you know it you will be in love with your body in its entirety ... well, maybe almost all its entirety!

CULTIVATING SENSUALITY

Sensuality is the art of feeling energy through the skin. It's a delicious art and one that we often ignore. Our skin is incredibly sensitive and, with a little gentle training, can become more sensitive yet. Begin your exploration by noticing how different temperatures and textures feel on your skin. Start indoors, undress and lie on different surfaces – feel, really feel, how wood feels; how carpet feels; how wool feels different from leather or suede. Experiment with velvet, silk, fur (real on a cat; fake on a throw – what's the difference?) Notice how each surface makes you feel. See if you can detect the energy of the different materials. Does the real wood feel different from the synthetic rug? How does stone feel different to vinyl? Extend your senses – become aware. Take notice.

Explore water – feel the difference between the energy of the sea and that of a lake; between a swimming pool and a fast-running stream.

When you have explored your house with your senses on full alert, go outside and do the same. Take off as many clothes as you can and lie on the grass, on the sand or pebbles of the beach, on the leaves of the forest. Explore water – feel the difference between the energy of the sea and that of a lake; between a swimming pool and a fast-running stream.
All these exercises will serve you well in other areas of your energywork. We will certainly revisit them when we look at nature energy.

As you learn to feel through your skin you may be surprised by what you learn. With your new-found sensitivity explore what your body really likes and wants. Does it like a firm touch or a gentle one? If you are lucky enough to live in an area with a variety of bodyworkers (and the money to afford massage) try out different forms – from the gentle soothing strokes of aromatherapy massage to the vigorous pummelling of Swedish massage. See whether you prefer the almost imperceptible touch of Reiki or the strong stretching of Thai massage or Shiatsu. What does each do for your energy?

PLAYING WITH SENSUAL ENERGY

If you have a partner, now is the time to start working with each other. Before you can start working with pure sexual energy you need to be able to connect on an energetic level. This is why we have spent a fair amount of time first working on ourselves, becoming attuned to our own sensual energy. Only once we know how to direct and connect with our own energy can we go further into exchanging energy with someone else.

So, before you launch into sex, you need to spend some time building trust and playing with each other's energy.

Start with these simple exercises. They teach us how to work together and, if you perform them mindfully, you should be able to sense your partner's energy and your own.

CONNECTING WITH THE BREATH

1. Sit down in front of each other in whatever position you feel comfortable.

2. Just sit quietly for a few minutes, focusing on your own breathing. Keep your eyes cast down into your lap.

3. When you both feel centred and comfortable, raise your eyes and gently, softly, make eye contact. Don't stare and don't feel you can't break eye contact. Just really look at that person.

4. Notice how they are breathing. Is it slower or faster than your own breathing? Make a slight shift so you come more into tune with their breathing. How do you feel? Of course, the other person will be doing the same to you so you should settle into a form that is halfway between the two of you. Again, don't force it and don't make yourself uncomfortable. Just see if there is a breath which suits both of you and sense how it feels to breathe together, to share the same breath.

5. Continue the connection by gently holding hands. Imagine the energy flowing in and around the two of you. You may well feel the tingling of energy in your fingertips. Experiment by holding up your hands, palms facing each other, about two inches apart. You may feel a pull, as if you were two magnets. Try moving your hands further apart and then closer together. How does the energy change?

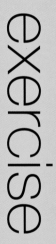

exercise

exercise

THE SEE-SAW

This yoga exercise helps to build trust with your partner. It is also very energizing and helps mobilize the body.

1. Sit down facing your partner.

2. Both of you stretch out your legs as wide as feels comfortable. Touch each other's toes so your legs form a diamond shape.

3. Reach out to clasp each other's hands or fingers. If you can reach, hold each other's wrists. You may need to bend your knees slightly in order to touch.

4. Start to gently sway forwards and backwards – one partner leans back while the other bends forward.

5. Breathe – try inhaling as you lean forward and exhaling as you lean back. Smile at each other.

6. After a few minutes, stop swaying and slowly separate your hands and bring your legs back together.

7. Now sit back to back with your eyes closed for a few moments. Try to connect once more with each other's breath.

BACK BENDS

Again, this is a wonderful exercise in trust. You have to rely, quite literally, on your partner. The deep stretching stimulates energy and makes your body more flexible and relaxed.

1. Both of you should sit down, back to back. You can either stretch out your legs in front of you or have them crossed – whichever feels most comfortable. Link your arms together.

2. One of you leans gently forward, pulling the other so his or her back is stretched over yours. Keep the movement slow and even – don't jerk and don't stretch further than is comfortable for your partner. Then reverse the movement so the other is 'stretched'.

3. Continue stretching back and forwards in a smooth, gentle rhythm for as long as you like. Check to make sure you are relaxing your whole body – then you will be able to stretch even deeper. Keep breathing as you do this.

SENSUAL MASSAGE

Giving your partner a massage – whether a gentle foot rub or a sensual full body massage – is an ideal way to foster intimacy and to gently stimulate your sensual energy. You don't need to be an expert – far from it. There are plenty of books and videos showing you how to perform massage or you can simply follow your intuition, and listen to your partner's feedback. Be very respectful and always remember that we are all different. While you might adore rough, tough bodywork (yes, some people even like Rolfing!) your partner might have a very low pain threshold and prefer something a lot gentler. Generally speaking, when you are performing a sensual massage you won't want anything too strenuous – or the effect will be more boot-camp than boudoir!

Here are some basic guidelines for sensual massage – but do be guided by your intuition and your energy and that of your partner.

1. Make the environment as inviting as possible. The room should be pleasantly warm. Light candles and put on some relaxing music in the background. You may like to burn some sensual oil (such as sandalwood or ylang-ylang) in a burner.

2. Make up your massage oil. Use six drops of either ylang-ylang or sandalwood oil in 4 teaspoons (15–20ml) of a base oil such as sweet almond.

3. You don't have to be an expert in massage – just remember to keep a slow, steady rhythm with the right amount of pressure for your partner.

4. Start on the back with your thumbs on either side of the spine, fingers pointing towards the neck. Allow your hands to glide slowly up the body and around the shoulders. Draw your hands lightly down the side of the back to your starting position.

5. Fleshy areas such as hips and thighs can be kneaded gently – lift, squeeze and roll the skin between the thumb and fingers of one hand and glide it towards the other hand.

6. Curl your fingers into loose fists, keeping the fingers (not the knuckles) against the skin. Work all over the body.

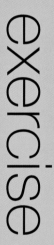

exercise

7. Make small circling movements on the shoulders, palms of the hands, soles of the feet and chest.

8. Form your hands into cup shapes and with quick, light movements move over the skin as if you were beating a drum.

9. Ask your partner to turn over and continue your massage on his or her front. Stroke the inner thighs, gently trace your fingers over the belly. Circle the nipples. Be teasing – gently touch the genitals as if by accident!

10. Be inventive. Towards the end of your massage you could use your whole body to massage your partner – or trail your hair over their body. Try also lightly scratching – as if you were a large cat.

11. As you reach the end of your sensual massage you want to wake your partner up so use light pummelling – put your hands into loose fists and lightly bounce the side of the hands alternately against the skin.

SACRED SEXUALITY

This is the point where we move from sensuality to sexuality. Having mindful, sacred sex can be quite confrontational so don't be surprised if you find it hard to make the next step. In our society we have become adept at divorcing ourselves from our bodies and nowhere more so than in the sexual act: a huge number of people have been brought up to think of sex as something smutty, dirty and unclean. Take a moment to think about how you feel about sex.

● How were you brought up to think about sex?

● Was it openly discussed in your household – or was it kept quiet and secret?

● What were your early experiences of sexuality? When did you first masturbate? How did you feel? Did you and your friends or siblings experiment with yourselves and each other? Did you see or hear any adults having sex? How did that make you feel?

● Do you remember your first kiss? Your first sexual encounter? How was it and how did you feel?

● Think about your sexual relationships? Have they been similar in any ways?

● Are you happy with your sex life? Your sexuality? Is there anything you do in bed you don't feel happy with? What do you like? What would you change?

Ask your partner to think about these questions too. Discuss them. They can form the basis for an open and enlightening conversation. You might find that neither of you is happy with your sex life but you both thought the other was OK. You may find you have more in common than you thought. Sex is something we rarely discuss, even with our sexual partners! Use your new-found knowledge to shift your lovemaking. Start by becoming more aware of what you do and how you feel. Explore your partner's body as if you had never seen it before. Really investigate it and notice everything, from the lobes of their ears to their little toes.
Don't just pounce on each other – take it slowly. Use your freshly-awakened sensual energy to detect the nuances of skin touching skin. Feel the texture of your partner's body. Use your hair, your nails, your eyelashes (!) to stroke his or her body. Find out what each of you really loves. If you're not sure, ask.

Rediscover the lost art of kissing. When you're an adolescent there is nothing more mysterious and arcane, yet when we grow up kissing often gets passed over. Try every kind of kiss you can imagine – wherever you can imagine.

Animal sexuality

Imagine your sexual energy expresses itself as an animal – what would it be? Would you be a slinky panther or a sinuous snake? A playful chimpanzee or a powerful bear? Act out your animal's energy and see if your partner can guess what you are. You might find you are two of a pair – or you might have very different animals. Take it in turns and try to tune in to the animal energy of your partner, as well as your own. Make love as if you were those animals – keeping within what feels good for you both. Let go and become that animal – borrow its movements, its noises, its expressions. Or be more subtle and make love with the energy of that animal.

Uncovering the wild man and wild woman inside

Another way to unleash our primal sexual energy is to rediscover the wilderness within. In every ancient culture there are gods and goddesses who are considered 'wild', untamed, unfettered, free. Their energy is primal, raw and frequently sexual in nature – sex is one of our earliest, most basic needs. There is also a lot of humour there too. Think about Baubo, the strange little Greek goddess whose eyes are in her breasts and whose mouth is in her vagina. She tells bawdy stories and ribald jokes. Then there's Pan, the priapic God with the huge erect penis, which always leads him into trouble. Baubo and Pan teach us not to take ourselves, or even sex, too seriously. Find a place for their humour in your bedroom.

Most of the ancient male gods have powerful sexual energy. Many female goddesses are also sexually powerful. Modern women desperately need to re-discover their inner 'wild woman'. So read up the stories of the wild goddesses – Kali, Sekhmet, Medusa, Erishkegal. Meditate on them and conjure their wildness into your sex play.

Elemental sex

Make use of the elements within sex. Feel the differing energies of fire, wind, water, air and earth, and play with incorporating them into your lovemaking. Imagine you are made of the earth, take on its steady, deep, throbbing energy. Touch each other as lightly as the air itself. Be playful, like the wind, surprising, unpredictable. Then feel the fire energy, flickering over your body, scorching your lips, tingling your penis, your vulva, lapping like a small, persistent tongue. And, as you become more aroused, feel the water energy mounting up within in, rolling and thundering like huge breakers as it subsumes your entire body in its embrace.

RAISING ENERGY WITH TANTRA

Aside from the mystical joining of male and female forces during lovemaking, Tantrics aim to unite the male and female forces within their own bodies. In fact, some modern schools of Tantric yoga do not use physical sex at all, but concentrate on this more esoteric union. The practice is called 'raising Kundalini'. Kundalini is the fire serpent supposed to lie coiled in the base of the spine. It is the material manifestation of the divine female energy of the goddess Shakti. In most of us, Kundalini lies quietly slumbering, quite unaware that way up in our heads is her divine counterpart Shiva. Exercises involving visualization and rhythmic contraction of the anal sphincter are supposed to 'wake' Kundalini who will then start to ascend through the chakras right up to the head where she will join in ecstatic union with Shiva. The result is supposedly a vast surge of energy and a huge sense of well-being. However, most Tantric teachers say it is not advisable to attempt to wake Kundalini until you are quite far along the mystic path. So I am not going to explain precisely how to raise Kundalini here.

THE SACRED RITUAL OF TANTRA

The full sacred ritual of Tantric sex is known as panchatattva, with the mystical union itself known as maithuna. In Tantric schools this is a very precise ritual, not allied to sexual pleasure at all. It is a form of worship – the male energy and female energy joining together, Shiva and Shakti returning to their divine congress. However, I don't feel that should put us lesser mortals off trying it. I have found that even this simplified version can have quite extraordinary effects – unlike anything usually experienced in sex.

One point that is worth mentioning is the question of same sex partners. The Tantric texts all refer to maithuna being carried out between a man and a woman, but I do not see why, if you are confident with sensing energy, you should not practise a version of maithuna with your same-sex partner. What is important in this ritual is the polarity of energies. One of you should decide to take on the masculine Shiva energy; the other the feminine Shakti energy. For the sake of ease, I shall describe the ritual in the traditional different-sex version.

exercise

Now you're ready to progress to the full Tantric ritual, make the whole experience really special. Decide in advance when you are going to hold your rite and plan every detail. Your room should be spotlessly clean, with fresh sheets and exotic coverings over the bed. Try to shut out the outside world: pull the curtains shut or pin coverings over windows.

Soft background music should be playing and you should have fresh flowers around the room – traditionally these would be red. Burn either incense (musk, patchouli or sandalwood work well) or essential oils (ylang ylang and sandalwood are traditional choices but pick those you both like). Candles, traditionally red again, provide soft sensual lighting.

Prepare some food in advance. Traditionally, Tantrics ate food they weren't accustomed to, or foods that were taboo, in order to jolt their consciousness into a different realm. But you don't have to carry it that far. Make a careful choice of light, tasty nibbles and lay them on a china plate on a silver tray. Include, if you can, fish, meat, cereal and fruit. Traditionally there would be wine and water scented with a few drops of rose water. Cardomoms would be sprinkled on the tray so you could sweetly scent your breath.

When everything is ready you should both take a bath or shower. As you take off your clothes, imagine you are dropping off your everyday persona. As you bathe, imagine all the dross of the day being washed away. As you step out of the bath imagine you are taking on the attributes of the God and Goddess. You are Shakti, the embodiment of female energy. You are Shiva, embodiment of male energy. Anoint your body with delicate scent – musk for Shakti, patchouli for Shiva. Dress in a loose comfortable robe of red silk or linen.

Now both of you should sit quietly. Face each other and follow each other's breathing. When you feel comfortable, shift to a new pattern of breathing: breathe in to the count of seven, hold for one count and then exhale for seven. Repeat this 12 times. As you inhale for the thirteenth time, hold your breath for seven counts before exhaling for seven. While you hold your breath, focus your attention on the base chakra. Contract your anus and imagine the divine union of Shakti and Shiva. As they join together, a stream of energy flows up from the base of your spine to your head.

exercise

Bring your breathing back to normal and eat and drink the food, wine and water. Do not overdo the wine! Bring consciousness to your eating – as we did in Part One. Lastly, eat the cardomoms to sweeten your breath. Now spend some time just gently gazing at each other. Try to invest each other with the attributes of the Goddess and God. See and feel the divine power you each have within you. Wonder at it, be awed by it. Take it in turns to anoint each other. Use the index and middle fingers of the right hand to touch the following parts of your partner's body in turn: the heart; the crown of the head; the eyelids; the third eye; the hollow of the throat; the ear lobes; the breasts; the upper arms; the navel; the thighs; the knees and the penis or vulva (known in Tantra as the lingam and yoni).

Shiva should now meditate on the image of the vulva, the yoni, picturing it as warm, welcoming, moist and soft, opening and closing like a flower. He should concentrate on the soft smell of musk and imagine the sound of a heartbeat. Meanwhile Shakti meditates on the penis, the lingam, visualizing it as erect and swollen, mentally examining its different textures. The scent to imagine is of the tiniest sea-side smell of seminal fluid, or the scent of patchouli. The sound is a faster, more insistent throb. Shiva and Shakti now move close together. Shakti brings Shiva's lingam into her deeply and solidly. Any position can be used but many prefer sitting face to face. For a while just move slowly, the woman milking (contracting her vaginal muscles) and the man thrusting gently. Then become totally still, staring deep into each other's eyes. Imagine yourselves linked at the various chakras, or power centres of the body: at the head, the throat, the heart, the solar plexus and particularly the genitals.

Imagine your genitals surrounded by a pulsing orb of deep red light. Now synchronize your breathing, slowly and deeply breathing towards your partner's mouth. Then imagine the energy generated from your genitals spreading up your spines and throughout your entire bodies. Stay in this position for as long as is comfortable. If the man feels he is coming close to ejaculation he should hold his breath and turn his tongue backwards as far as possible against the roof of his mouth.

Ideally you would stay like this – immobile, in perfect union, for thirty-two minutes. You would not experience ejaculation or a clitoral orgasm but, instead, a total body orgasm which is known as samarasa and an incredible feeling of love and unity. But don't worry if you can't get even close to that. Even if you manage a few minutes, it should still result in an unusual experience for you and your partner.

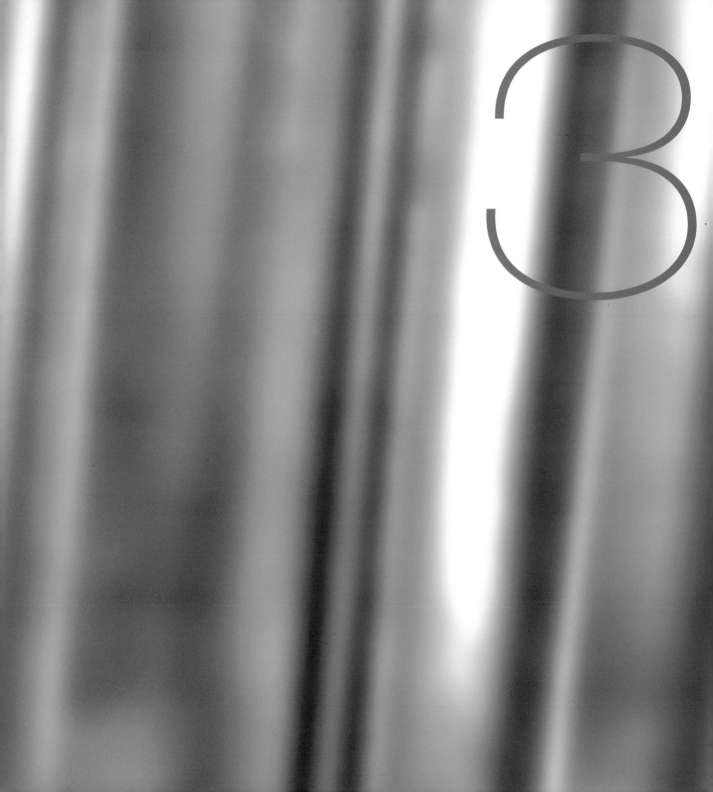

environmental**energy**

CHAPTER EIGHT

THE ENERGY OF THE HOME

Homes have an energy all of their own. Some places you walk into and feel a sense of well-being and relaxation. Other places have a frenzied, anxious atmosphere, which makes you feel harried and unsettled. Yet more places feel full of foreboding, as if they were filled with an unpleasant psychic energy. Most lie somewhere in the middle. Once you understand the concept of vital energy these differences make sense. As we've already discussed, energy can flow smoothly or it can become stuck and clogged. Just as we humans need to keep our internal energy moving in the optimum manner, so energy in buildings needs to flow smoothly. Yet here in the West, hardly anyone knows how to sense and move energy. So we live in the psychic equivalent of dustbins – in homes full of age-old stagnant energy. The very fabric of the house soaks up the energy of the people who live in it – so some very old houses could be full of literally centuries of arguments, bad moods and unpleasant emotions!

Some places you walk into and feel a sense of well-being and relaxation. Other places have a frenzied, anxious atmosphere, which makes you feel harried and unsettled.

Most of us are sensitive to the energy in houses, to one degree or another. We've all had the experience of walking into a room and being able to 'cut the air with a knife' because there has recently been an unpleasant argument. We all have places in which we feel safe and serene – and others in which we feel uncomfortable and edgy. The aim of working with home energy is to be able to shift the mood of any room in which you have to spend time. You can cleanse your home of any old unpleasant atmospheres and claim it as your own. This is particularly useful when you move into a new home – the place will be full of the vibrations of the last inhabitants (unless of course they were energy-workers!) You need to politely but firmly move their energy on and install your own. I also firmly believe that when you move out of a house or apartment it's only good manners to clear the energy and leave it clear and clean for the next inhabitants. You wouldn't leave a place physically dirty – so why should you leave your psychic mess?

Of course other, wiser, cultures have a long, venerable tradition of space clearing and cleansing. The Chinese system of feng shui, the Indian vastu shastra, the Native American smudge ceremony, the Balinese bell-ringing and flower-offering ceremonies are all ways of shifting energy in the home. Let's try to reclaim the lost art of energy sensing here in the West!

exercise

SENSING THE ENERGY OF YOUR HOME

Before you try any energy-shifting work in your home you need to attune yourself to the energy of your home as it stands. Prepare yourself by taking off your shoes and any jewellery.

● Sit down quietly and centre yourself by consciously becoming aware of your breath. Gently shut your eyes.

● Connect with the chakras – feel the base chakra connecting you to the Earth; the crown chakra linking you with the cosmic energy of the Universe. Feel your solar plexus chakra, the centre of your body, uniting the two.

● Breathe into your solar plexus, quietly feeling the strength and purpose of this chakra radiating out through your body. Your energy is moving from inside you to quest outside. It is as if it were putting out feelers, gauging the energy of your home.

● Let your solar plexus, your 'gut reaction', tell you where the energetic centre of your home lies. It may be in the physical centre of the house but equally it might be somewhere else.

● How does the energy feel in your home? What sense do you get from it? Is it calm or a bit frenzied? Does it feel stuck in any places? What word would you use for the energy in your home? If your home were to have a secret name what would it be?

● Now go to the centre of the home and honour this spot. Light a candle, burn some incense, make contact with the energy of your home. Ask your home what it would like from you.

When you take the time to tune in to your home you might gain some surprising insights. You could suddenly realize that you need more fun/more peace/more serenity in your life. You might gain a sudden inspiration and 'see' the perfect colour to decorate your living room.

DECLUTTERING AND CLEANSING

One thing you might notice is that you need to have a clear-out. As we already know, energy likes to flow in smooth lines. If it comes across a pile of clutter it becomes stuck, like dust in a corner. If it isn't cleared, the stuck energy attracts more energy and you end up with a nasty pile of clutter surrounded by a 'pile' of stagnant energy. Things will start to go wrong in your life – you will feel 'stuck' and frustrated. Money may be slow to come in. Surely more than enough reasons to get rid of those piles of newspapers and heaps of dirty clothes!

ACTION PLAN FOR DECLUTTERING

● Decide how best you can declutter. Some people like to set aside a whole day and blitz through it; others cope better with sorting out a little at a time. If you're the former, make it a special day. Dress in work clothes, put on some inspiring music and make up a good pot of coffee. If you're the latter type of person, make a contract with yourself (say, half an hour a day – or a cupboard/drawer a day) and stick to it.

● Have a series of trash bags or boxes ready. One for absolute trash; one for things that belong to other people; one for things which can be sold/recycled/given to charity.

● Now go through each room systematically. First, clear the obvious mess. But then look beyond that. Do you really need all those clothes? Do you need every book that is cramming your bookshelves? Bookshelves should always have some gaps to welcome in new knowledge. Remember that you can always borrow books from libraries or look up information on the Internet.

● Hoarding is very bad energywork. The energy of the Universe seems to delight in free exchange. So if you are miserly with things and hoard, you are almost telling the Universe that you don't need anything else. Allowing things to flow from you makes space for new things to flow into your life.

● An essential tip: once you've sorted out your clutter, get rid of it IMMEDIATELY. Don't be tempted to keep it hanging around in bags or boxes because before you know it you will have grabbed something out and then another thing, or the bags and boxes themselves will just become more clutter.

● If you have loads of stuff belonging to other people, give them a deadline to claim it. Be very firm – tell them that if it hasn't gone within a reasonable time frame it will be given to charity.

● Once your house is free of all extraneous clutter, give it a good spring-clean. Open all the doors and windows and let the fresh air in while you work. Use non-toxic cleaning materials (I like to add a few drops of essential oils). Do some powerful housework magic – get down on your hands and knees and scrub the floors. As you do imagine you are scrubbing away all the old negative energy – leaving the place sparkling clean and ready to welcome in the new positive vibrations.

exercise

There is nothing that upsets the smooth flowing of

energy in the home as much as clutter

CLEARING TECHNIQUES

Once your house is clean and clutter-free you have a clear space with which to work. You need to get rid of any old, negative energy and then usher in the new. Every ancient wisdom culture has ceremonies and techniques for shifting energy – it is just us in the so-called 'civilized' West who have forgotten how to do it. Yet even we have vestiges of memory: the bells that ring out on Sundays and for weddings are cleansing the air with sound; incense in a church or in our homes is cleansing with the air element. When we have the urge to spring-clean after the winter we are following our old deeply-ingrained instincts. But for really effective cleansing we need to consult the experts – cultures such as the Balinese, the Native Americans, the Indians, Chinese and Tibetans. The following techniques come from a variety of sources. You can use them all or pick the ones that appeal to you. Of course, you are also free to shift or alter them as your intuition demands – a vital part of cultivating your own energy.

Before you start any of these exercises spend some time readying yourself. Take a shower or have a bath (you need to be clean too!) – add a couple of drops of bergamot or lemon essential oil. Dress in clean, comfortable clothes but leave your feet bare and don't wear any jewellery or a watch. Stand in the energetic centre of your home and centre yourself. The bubble of light exercise on page 91 is a very useful way to cleanse your own energy in preparation. If you have any spirit guardians (guardian angels, or a power animal) you may like to ask their help.

● **CLAPPING**. Work systematically around the corners of each room. You start with your hands low down facing towards the floor and then clap several times as you move your arms upwards until you are clapping towards the ceiling. At first the sound may be dull but as you repeat your clapping it should become clearer. Keep going until the sound becomes clear. Make sure you clap out each corner – including alcoves – energy gets most stuck in corners.

● **SMUDGING.** Smudging is a form of cleansing that comes from the Native American tradition. You can buy smudge sticks (bundles of sacred herbs – traditionally sagebrush, cedar and sweetgrass) from New Age shops or you can make your own. You simply need to bind together 12-inch (roughly) lengths of the herbs and leave them until almost dry. Rosemary, lavender and culinary sage are alternatives. All the herbs used in smudging are considered sacred, with the power to banish negative energy and attract the positive. Light your smudge stick and blow on it until it is smoking well (but not flaming). Fan the smoke around you – to cleanse your aura –

ending by directing it towards your heart and solar plexus chakras. Then take the smudge stick and send smoke into each corner of the room plus the centre. Ask the sacred spirits of the plants to take away all negativity and replace it with beneficial, healing energy. Make sure you thank the spirits when you have completed your work. Incense can also cleanse energy in a similar way. Choose a scent you like and to which your intuition has guided you. You can direct the smoke as with a smudge stick or leave one burning in each room. Note: this is not as powerful as smudging and is better combined with other techniques.

● **SOUND CLEANSING:** Many cultures use bells, rattles, drums and other sounds to cleanse the air. If you have one of these instruments with a particularly resonant sound you can use that in your rituals. Again, centre yourself and ask the instrument's spirit to help you in your cleansing. Beat, rattle or ring as you go around the home, imagining all the negativity being driven away by the healing sound. If you don't have an instrument you can always use your own voice. The chakra toning exercise on page 26 is very cleansing. Once you have cleared your own chakras with it you can direct the sound out into the home. A house is just like a body and has chakras or energy centres, just like us. So resonate the base chakra into the foundations of your house. The crown with the roof. Use your imagination and intuition to detect where the other chakras lie in your home. The kitchen might be the solar plexus – or it could be the heart of your home where everyone gathers. Where would be the throat chakra, the centre for communication? The front door perhaps – or the room with the computer or the phone?

FENG SHUI AND VASTU SHASTRA – COSMIC ENERGY IN THE HOME

In countries such as China and India buildings were situated according to precise energetic rules. In China the science of placement is known as feng shui; in India as vastu shastra – both are very stringent about where one should build and where one should not. While virtually everyone in the West now knows about feng shui, vastu is less well-known.
The theory in both systems is the same. When energy (chi in Chinese, prana in Indian) is well-regulated and smooth running in a house, the lives of the inhabitants will run smoothly too. Feng shui and vastu shastra are both very complex sciences, based on many thousands of years of energy observation. There is not space in a book this size to go into them in huge detail – once again, I would suggest you read *Spirit of the Home* or one of the books in the bibliography for more detail. However, there are certain things anyone can do with no detailed knowledge of either system to get the energy moving smoothly. Try these:

SIMPLE HOME ENERGIZERS AND HARMONIZERS

● **USE IONIZERS:** Everyone knows how good you feel by the ocean or out in the countryside where the air is negatively charged. Positive ions, which build up in houses and cities make us feel tired and irritable. Ionizers keep your air negatively charged, or keep bowls of fresh water in rooms to absorb positive ions.

● **NAME YOUR HOUSE:** Naming your house helps to give it personality; it links it with you and your energetic fortune. Use your intuition to pick a name that suits both you and the house. You may find it has two – its 'outer' name and its 'secret' name, which outlines its underlying energy.

● **USE THE POWER OF SCENT:** Aromatherapy oils can make a house feel brighter or create an atmosphere of calm and tranquillity. Try peppermint or lemongrass for an uplifting effect or sandalwood and lavender for relaxation. Tea tree is strongly anti-viral and anti-bacterial. Geranium is a cheering, happy oil. The citrus oils are refreshing and uplifting.

● **ALLOW SOUND INTO YOUR HOME:** Feng shui uses wind-chimes as a cure for problems, but even if you don't specifically need them it can be lovely to hear the soft sound of chimes. The sound of water is soothing and energizing too. Think about having an interesting water feature either inside or outside. If you have young children pick one where water runs over large pebbles or a boulder so toddlers can't fall in.

● **HAVE LIFE IN YOUR HOUSE:** Feng shui practitioners say that live creatures and plants bring energy into your home. If you work on a computer your best friend will be a spider plant: they soak up radiation and ionize the air. Animals introduce plenty of energy into houses – but you don't need to cope with a large dog or even a cat – in feng shui goldfish are valued very highly. Ideally, have eight red fish and one black in your bowl – and keep the water fresh with an aerator.

● **CHOOSE WELL-CRAFTED PRODUCTS:** Originally created arts and crafts have much more energy than mass-created items. Natural materials (wood, stone, ceramic, metal, natural fibres such as cotton, linen, wool) have much more energy than 'dead' synthetics. Items that please your soul will infuse your home with vibrant, soulful energy.

● **KEEP YOUR HOUSE FULL OF FLOWERS:** Fresh flowers bring a wonderful energy into the home. You don't have to spend a fortune on shop-bought bouquets – branches in bud or bloom look wonderful. Pick armfuls of 'weeds'. Grow wheatgrass or reclaim a bit of childhood and grow cress on blotting paper.

BRINGING COLOUR INTO YOUR HOME

One of the simplest ways of changing the energy in your home is to use colour. It doesn't have to be a complete redecoration – you can introduce splashes of colour to energize particular corners. Intuition counts for a lot – what colours feel right? The following gives a few ideas on colour to get you started but don't take them as a rigorous prescription.

Think in terms of the chakras again. Vibrant reds and oranges relate to the lower chakras and work best in downstairs rooms. Yellow is a good downstairs colour, which can also be an intermediary between the levels. Green bridges the two floors. Blues are great for bedrooms and bathrooms. Violets and indigos are fine for bedrooms and even better for top floor meditation or relaxation rooms.

● **Red** is the great energizer. It is a lucky colour in feng shui, but be careful not to overdo it or it becomes overpowering. Red is linked with power, passion, energy and challenge. It will help keep you alert but can be tiring. Use it for rooms with lots of activity. A few red pillows and a red throw can help promote passion in the bedroom.

● **Orange** promotes joy and brings confidence and sociability. Again, this is a very powerful colour, which needs handling with care. It stimulates the appetite so avoid it if you're on a diet! Use it in rooms you use for entertaining.

● **Yellow** lifts the spirits and raises your energy levels. It works brilliantly in many rooms of the house, bringing joyful energy to kitchens, living rooms, hallways and bathrooms. It's also ideal for home studies and workrooms as it stimulates the left side of the brain, which governs logic.

● **Green** is the great balancer. The colour of nature, it is soothing and calming. Green is considered a very lucky colour in feng shui. It is reassuring and harmonious – use it if you need to soothe the energy of your home. It's particularly useful for troubled teenagers.

● **Blue** promotes relaxation and peace. It's supremely restful but also promotes good communication. Use soft blue in bedrooms to ensure a good night's rest. It's also a good colour for a home office if you need to communicate a lot in your work.

● **Indigo** is the colour of the third eye. In its pure form it is too intense for anything other than the odd bolt of colour, but, toned down to a soft shade, it works well for a bedroom or meditation retreat. Light shades of violet and lavender are soothing for bedrooms and healing spaces.

BALANCING YOUR HOME'S ENERGY WITH THE ELEMENTS

Another lovely way to harmonize the flow of natural energy within the home is to ensure we incorporate all the elements – fire, air, water and earth. All ancient cultures understood the need for balance between the elements and took care to ensure that their homes contained representations of all of them. Before you start, take a moment to think about your home once again. If it were an element, which would it be? Do you live in a passionate fire home or a cool cerebral air home? Is yours an emotional water home or a practical, down-to-earth earth home? You can often tell by the colours to which you are drawn – earthy homes are usually filled with muted browns, taupes and fawn, splashes of terracotta and brick red. Fire homes are bright and vivid – red is an obvious favourite, but anything colourful and vibrant attracts fire. Watery homes are filled with the colours of the sea and the riverbed – often very artistic homes with lots of paintings, paint effects and the dreaded clutter! Air homes are the ones you often see in magazines, clean, airy, spacious, often minimalist and slightly cool. Of course your home could be a combination of any or all of these – and if it is then you probably have a pretty balanced life. If you fall directly into one category though it may be worth introducing some other elements.

Here are some thoughts to get you started on your elemental voyage.

FIRE – The Energizer

Fire has been used to bring energy, spirit and soul to the home in every culture since the very beginning of humankind. The original heart of every home was the hearth, the living flame – in the past it was honoured as a deity in its own right and when a young woman married her mother would bring fire from her own hearth to that of her daughter. The fire would be lit and the young woman would now be mistress of her own home and guardian of its energy.

Fire ushers fresh vibrant energy into the house. If you can have a real fire in your home do so. A fire can bring warmth, strength and a feeling of peace. Roast chestnuts on it, cook toast or crumpets. Or just gaze into its flickering depths and see if you can see the salamanders – the spirits of fire.

If you cannot have a real fire, bring the fire element into your home with candles. Candle magic is a very ancient, very simple, yet very effective skill. First choose a colour that suits your purpose. Blue will help you achieve peacefulness and balance; reds or yellow will bring lively energy. If you are seeking love or wish to conceive a child, burn a pink candle in your bedroom. A green candle is helpful for money and abundance. Yellow candles can bring joy and conviviality. To gain the maximum benefit you need first to focus your intention, so that before you light the candle you are very clear as to why you are lighting it. Then concentrate intensely while lighting the candle. You could also write your wish on the candle – and watch your intent burn, sending your desire up into the ether where it can be transformed into manifestation. Sometimes, of course, dreams aren't supposed to come true! I once did some candle magic to attract the love of a man. I wrote his name on the candle but, to my dismay, as the candle burned the strip with his name on it did not. I was left with a small strip of wax rolled up with his name still on it. Obviously that was a relationship that was never meant to be! Also, hanging cut-lead crystals in your windows will help to bring the fire energy of the sun into your home. Children, in particular, love the rainbows that dance round the room from crystals. So do cats: my usually very dignified black cat turns into a kitten careering and leaping when the beams skitter around the walls. Try as well to hang mirrors in strategic places so that the sunshine can be reflected into your home.

WATER – The Purifier

Water, the next element, has a wonderful purifying energy and has been used in spiritual ceremonies since ancient times right up to modern baptism services. Water is excellent for clearing a room of negative emotions. After an argument, the air in a room might seem thick and almost charged with negative energy. The fastest way to neutralize this residual energy is to mist the room. The fine spray also creates a negative-ion-rich environment – such as you find next to a waterfall, or by the sea or in a pine forest.

The key is to use spring water in a fine spray – lightly spray all over the room. You can also use the Bach flower remedies in a mister – maybe Rescue Remedy after an argument or illness; Cherry Plum for calm, quiet courage; Star of Bethlehem to clear tension; Water Violet for tranquillity, poise and grace. Or check out the full list on page 40.

Equally you could try combining aromatherapy with misting. Add a drop (no more) of essential oil to the misting water. Use lemon or grapefruit in the kitchen; geranium or bergamot in the living room and lavender or sandalwood in the bedroom.

AIR – The Transformer

While water heals, cleanses and rejuvenates, the element of air transforms. Air changes all that it encompasses. A simple way to enliven a room is to light a stick of incense. But choose a scent that you like and which feels appropriate for the room. Aromatherapy can also be powerful medicine for the home. Our bodies react emotionally and powerfully to different scents and the smells in your home can contribute to or detract greatly from the way you feel about it. Use oils in vaporizers or diffusers, in a bowl of hot water or onto a ring that fits on your light bulb. Try the following: orange, lemon and grapefruit are uplifting and refreshing; geranium balances mood swings; chamomile is excellent after an argument; pine is refreshing and cleansing; rosemary helps with studying. The following oils work well in combination: lavender, rose geranium and ylang ylang for the bedroom; rosemary, peppermint, basil and bergamot in the study; orange, mandarin and bergamot in the living room; lemon and grapefruit in the kitchen; peppermint and pine in the bathroom. (Note: be careful with essential oils if you are pregnant or suffer from epilepsy – consult an aromatherapist before using.)

Bring fresh air into the house whenever you can – open the windows every day if you can – even if only for a few minutes. Fans circulate air – old fashioned ceiling ones look great too. Air conditioning unfortunately does not have the same effect and can actually have the opposite effect. If you have to have air conditioning keep it on as little as possible.
A sense of air comes through space as well. Try to have at least one room in the house which has an airy quality – without too much furniture or objects. A room with freedom and possibilities, where your mind is free to roam unfettered. Such rooms are wonderful for children too – they can move freely in the wild way they need, without fear of being told off for crashing into things or breaking things.

EARTH – The Strengthener

Earth is grounding and strengthening. It brings stability, ancient wisdom and power into our lives. Introducing earth into your home will generate an energy that is serene and stable. You will feel more certain of your direction in life. We all need a sense of earth in our homes – and particularly so if we live in upper floor apartments without firm foundations beneath our feet. Salt is one of the most powerful ways of bringing earth into the home. Salt has the ability to neutralize negativity and to cleanse the aura. It is a powerful purifier, in the ocean it acts as an antiseptic and it has been used in rituals for centuries – in the past church bells were anointed with salt and water to bless them. An ancient baptism ritual saw the baby rubbed with salt to repel demons. We still throw a pinch of salt over our shoulders to 'hit the devil in the eye'. If you ever feel as if you are being thrown off balance by outside influences, try the following. Take salt and make a large ring that goes around the periphery of your room, including all the corners. Then make a smaller circle of salt right around your bed. Just a small trickle will be effective.

Crystals and semi-precious stones can also help to bring earth into your home. Crystals act as catalysts and transformers for energy. They also look very beautiful. Pick your stones carefully – you will undoubtedly know which is 'your' stone – it's the one that calls your name! Before you place crystals or stones around your home you will need to cleanse them. Simply immerse the crystal in a bowl of water to which you have added a few pinches of sea salt. Leave it for 48 hours – ideally in the sunlight, then carefully dry it. It's a lovely idea to dedicate a stone as the 'house' crystal. Simply perform the chakra balancing technique (see page 26) then visualize pure energy coming down through your crown chakra into your heart chakra and from there into the crystal you are holding in your hands. Be clear about your intent – the stone could be to protect the house, to bring in warm loving energy, to guard a child's room or to foster good relationships.

The following stones can all be used in the home: citrine clears thoughts, promotes confidence, helps communication and decision-making; tiger's eye is grounding and focusing; rose quartz is excellent for helping children and family and also for aiding creativity and love; smoky quartz helps to promote wisdom and brings abundance; coral fosters physical strength and determination.

CHAPTER NINE

NATURAL ENERGY

How does the energy of a stone differ from that of a piece of wood? What does the river say as it flows past? Where are the secret shrines of the Earth Spirit? Few of us know anymore. We have become divorced from the natural world, from its ever-shifting, fluctuating energy. We seem to consider ourselves out of the loop. We hide away in our air-conditioned, centrally heated homes and rarely feel the cold breath of the north wind, the scorching heat of the noon-day sun. If we do go out we still tend to keep ourselves apart from Nature: we park our cars in picnic spots and sit on benches or portable chairs. If we go to the beach we lie on rugs. Rarely do we feel the grass or stone or sand under our feet. Rarely do we feel the wind in our hair or the rain on our skin.

What fools we are. Despite our attempts at taming it, it is still a beautiful world. Think of the dappled green of a forest with shafts of sunlight glancing through the trees; the rainbow shimmering through a waterfall; the awesome power of the mountains; the heaving fastness of the sea. And smaller beauties too: a fresh new bud; a butterfly alighting gently on a flower; a young puppy bounding with sheer joy.

Our ancestors would have laughed at the idea of having to search for the energy of the natural world. To them the world was their soul, just as they were the soul of the world – there was no distinction. Then came civilization and an awareness that here, on the one hand, stood us humans, while out there, apart from us, stood the world, foreign and dangerous. Our perspective changed: instead of feeling part of the natural world, we came to view ourselves as outside the natural world. Nature and its resources began to serve us, to be moulded to our needs and desires. Worse still, we began to almost 'punish' Nature, to put her 'in her place', to show our dominance and our superiority. It's as if we are trying to deny the fact that we are creatures like any others – we are born, we live and we die, according to Nature's rule. We can push back the clock but we can never stop it. So it seems almost an act of defiance to do our worst to Nature in a desperate attempt to prove that we can control the energy that, inevitably, inexorably, controls all of us.

There is a huge rift between us and the rest of Nature. If we want to reclaim our birthright as energy beings in an energetic world we have to do something to change this. The only true way to heal the rift is to accept, truly, that we are part of the great cycle of Nature, no more or less than the other denizens with whom we share this planet. Most of us live our lives cut

When we are cast adrift from earth energy we are dimly aware that something momentous, something intrinsic, is missing in our lives

adrift from earth energy, only dimly aware of a gap in our lives. We hark back to the 'good old days' when we perceived ourselves as being 'at one' with the land. We go to zoos to look at the animals, we take the children for a car-ride in 'the country' to 'look at Nature'. We delude ourselves that we are 'reconnecting with the land.' In fact, we are very very far away from that sense of energetic kinship.

We need to start, in the smallest of ways, to heal the rift: begin to sense the whole other world 'out there'. Try seeing everything – the grass, a bird, an insect, the earth – as if for the very first time. Don't just look – use your other senses too. Listen to the sounds of Nature. Go out and touch a tree, stroke a leaf, plunge your hands into the soil. Just begin to be aware of the world outside our houses, offices and cars. Start, just start, to think of yourself as part of this great cycle.

STONE AND LEAF ENERGY

Let's start small. Pick up a stone and a leaf. They don't have to be anything exceptional – any stone and leaf will do.

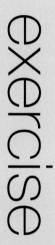

● Feel the weight and texture of the stone, its coolness perhaps. Sense its age. Imagine what it has quietly seen.

● How would it feel to be that stone? Take your time. What is 'stone energy' like? Try to feel its pulse, its rhythm.

● When you feel you know your stone, place it to one side and pick up the leaf instead. Feel the difference. Smell the difference.

● Trace the veins of your leaf. How would it feel to be a leaf, delicate yet attached to the strength and flexibility of a tree? How would it feel to have the sun falling on you; the sun you convert to energy and food? Imagine your life cycle as a leaf – concentrated inside a bud; then slowly pushing out into the sunlight; unfurling, growing, spreading; then slowly fading, drying, dying. Falling to the ground and slowly returning to the earth. It's a very different cycle to that of the stone. Keep your stone and leaf with you – perhaps on your desk or in a drawer.

exercise

LISTENING TO EARTH ENERGY

Another way of learning how to connect to earth energy is to Listen (with a capital L). This is so simple it sounds like child's play, but don't dismiss it for that – some of the greatest lessons we could learn are taught in kindergarten.

1. Find somewhere you can sit out in Nature, undisturbed. Ideally it will be somewhere in the country, but if that's not possible, take yourself into the garden or off to a local park. Sit on the ground and make yourself comfortable. Make sure you really are comfortable because this is not a speedy exercise. You need to give yourself at least 20 minutes.

2. Now close your eyes and start to breathe slowly and deeply. Let yourself become quiet, calm and centred. If invasive thoughts come up just gently let them drift away. Instead turn your attention to the world outside and start to listen. Just listen ... really listen.

3. At first you will probably hear nothing – or just invasive noises from far away. But before long you will start to tune in to the complex hum of Nature: the bewildering array of bird-calls; the scurrying of insects; the movement of leaves; the tentative progress of small creatures nosing through the undergrowth. As your hearing becomes more refined you will hear still more: a leaf dropping; a bud opening; the hum of the earth itself. That's when you begin to Listen.

4. If your thoughts start wandering off, gently pull them back to the listening. Don't beat yourself up about it; just accept it and quietly concentrate again.

5. You may feel uneasy or uncomfortable. Sometimes there is an incredibly powerful urge to open the eyes – particularly if you hear something strange or unexpected. Try to resist the urge and instead note the feeling, accept it and put it to one side. Time may become fluid – quite likely you won't be sure whether you have been listening for a few minutes or several hours. Don't worry about the disorientation, it's quite natural. If this worries you have a friend come with you as a 'guard'. Your friend can sit at a suitable distance away and can call you back after 20 minutes.

6. At the end of your time, write down what you heard and how you felt. Explore the feelings that came up – if you felt uncomfortable, can you work out why?

Once you've done this exercise once, it can become addictive. Not only does it attune your soul to the energy of the natural world but it also makes your sense of hearing more acute.

THE SHAMANIC PATH

There are people who can point the way back to living with earth energy. But we have to look in forgotten places, to those peoples who have been dismissed by the modern world. The indigenous cultures, the ancient 'primitive' ones, can teach us all lessons in finding our soul in the land. Chief Seattle, the Suquamish Native American leader put it beautifully:

'Whatever befalls the earth, befalls the sons and daughters of the earth. We did not weave the web of life; we are merely a strand of it. Whatever we do to the web, we do to ourselves.'

Think of a spider's web: even better, find one and watch. The web is intricate, a marvel of design. It has strength and flexibility, enough to withstand strong winds and harsh rain. Yet when an insect lands on the web even the tiniest contact sends out shock-waves through the whole web. The spider immediately knows something has happened. If a large insect inadvertently crashes through the web the whole shape and form of the web is shattered, it warps out of shape. The spider has to begin again.

Shamans say that the Spider weaves the web of Wyrd, or fate – an energy web that reaches all over the world, and out through the universe. We are all part of the web, what affects one part of the web will reverberate through and affect everything else. This is an idea that is echoed in the recent ideas of modern quantum physics and Chaos theory. But the spiders were there first. Watch them and wonder...

The Native Americans know this. So do the original Australians. In Bruce Chatwin's travelogue, *The Songlines*, he has explained to him the Aboriginal concept of the land. 'To wound the earth ... is to wound yourself, and if others wound the earth, they are wounding you.'
It's easy to think that such ideas are quaint and belong only to 'backward' peoples. But the idea of sacred earth energy was once prevalent all over the world.

Start, just start, to think of your connection with the whole world. Not just your tiny patch but the entire earth. Next time you see a TV documentary on some far-flung part of the world, remember that it is just another part of the web, your web.

The Medicine Path

Shamans remain close to the energy of the land. They watch for patterns in the web, seeing everything that happens in the natural world as having meaning, a resonance for our own personal energy field. Their training involves going out into Nature alone with the hope of contacting the spirits, the energy, of plants, animals, trees, the earth itself.

You can bring this awareness into your own hikes and even everyday life. Start by becoming aware of the natural world. Look at the trees – are they blowing in a particular way – what message might that have for you? A bird might fly in front of your car – what is the bird and what does its flight mean? A large pebble might plant itself in front of you as you walk to work. What message could there be there? There is no dictionary, no set interpretations – you have to follow your intuition here. What might it mean? If it had a meaning, what could it be? As you become more attuned to the energy around you, you will find that Nature can have many answers for you, much wisdom – if you only watch, listen and feel.

Most shamans develop special relationships with animals, birds, plants and even insects or reptiles. Some become 'allies', lending the shaman their particular energy or strengths. If you haven't already tried the exercise on page 135 for contacting the four great spirit animals, maybe now would be a good time. If you already have tried this, you could move on to finding your 'own' animal ally.

ANIMAL ENERGY

Choose a place – ideally outdoors – where you won't be disturbed. If the ground is dry and you can sit directly on the earth, so much the better. But if it's wet, don't risk piles for the sake of authenticity – sit on a groundsheet! If you like you can sit yourself within a medicine wheel – a circle of stones representing the various directions and their energies. You can construct a mini 'medicine wheel' by placing a stone in front of you, behind you, to the right and left of you, imagining they are being guarded by the great spirit animals, Eagle, Bear, Coyote and Buffalo. If you can't find stones, visualize them in place.

1. Start by following the listening exercise earlier in this chapter. Use it to become still and aware of the world around you.

2. When you feel very still and centred, and tuned in to the world directly around you, ask, very respectfully, if it is the right time for you to meet your guardian animal – your spirit ally. Keep your eyes gently closed and wait patiently.

3. You may 'see' an animal or bird. You might 'hear' it or just sense it. The image or name of one might pop into your head. Or nothing might happen at all. Be patient. Assure the animal world that you come in peace, with the desire to learn. Nature energy has become wary of humans (and quite rightly given our record in decimating the Earth).

4. If you do feel or sense an animal, ask its permission to speak to it. If it agrees, ask it if it is 'your' animal (or you are its human!) – whether it is willing to help you learn and share its energy with you. Be very respectful. If it agrees you can talk to it and ask its help and guidance. When you have finished, ask if there is anything you can do in return. Keep any promises you make.

5. Thank the animal. (Some people have fish or insect allies, though animals and birds are more usual.) It is customary to leave a little tobacco or cornmeal as an offering.

6. Come back to waking reality, stamp your feet and have something to eat or drink to ground you.

Once you have an animal ally, build on that relationship. You can call on your ally's energy when you need their strengths. For example, Eagle helps me on long car journeys, when I am feeling tired and not so sharp-sighted.

exercise

SACRED ENERGY

Every land has its sacred places – from the great mysterious sacred sites of antiquity to the quieter, more hidden spots that a stranger could easily pass by. These places – it could be a hill, a cave, a spring or a stone; or it could be a structure built or positioned by humans – a stone circle; a well; a church or a soaring menhir – seem to draw the soul like a magnet. They touch us in deep and unfathomable ways. These are places where the earth energy runs particularly strongly. Our ancestors, who could feel this energy, marked them as sacred and venerated the spirit of them, believing they were the residing places of gods, goddesses, spirits and elemental forces. If we take the time to stop and feel, to sense, we can often pick up on this. In fact, if you feel unsure about sensing natural energy you might find it easier if you go to one of these 'power' sources where the energy runs strong and can be more easily detected.

Our ancestors, who could feel this energy, marked them as sacred and venerated the spirit of them, believing they were the residing places of gods, goddesses, spirits and elemental forces.

As a child I had many favourite sacred spots. They ranged from the large 'public' sites, such as Glastonbury Tor and the Cerne Giant to tiny corners – a nook in a suburban wall where I left 'gifts' of flowers and stones and a forgotten corner by the railway track where I sat stock-still amongst the tall grass and tried to 'melt' into the earth. As I grew up and travelled I found more mysterious and powerful sacred spaces, full of the awe of earth energy. My soul shrank at first from the vastnesses of the desert in the South West of the USA – I felt like an ant, tiny and inconsequential. Then I took a deep breath and drank in the raw power and beauty of the place – the energy of rock and sky. I felt dizzy at the soaring mountains and endless forests of Wyoming and New Hampshire; then exhilarated by the clean, fresh air and the timeless splendor of tree and mountain. Stepping into the King's Chamber of the Great Pyramid at Giza was like being plugged directly into a battery, a source of superhuman spiritual power. But strangely, when I think about the places that resonated most with my own energy, they are neither the vast monuments nor the huge vistas: they are smaller, more personal spaces. There is a particular spring, hidden down a forgotten track, tucked away amidst trees and curling ivy. It is not large, or spectacular in any way, but it has a magic for me. I approach it as though visiting a lover, always mindful of taking it something – a daisy chain perhaps or a tiny posy of wild flowers tied with grass, maybe a little figure whittled from wood. Suddenly I'm there and I am overcome once again by its simple beauty. I sit on a rock and look into its bubbling waters. I give it my gift and watch it being swirled gently around in the ripples. I could stay there for hours, listening to the bird-song, simply watching the water. Like many springs it is said, by local legend, to have healing powers. You take a leaf from the overhanging tree, bend it into a cup and drink. As you drink, you also wish, but you must tell no-one your wish.

Of late 'my' well has become better-known and I have found litter by its banks, shouting voices splitting its peace. With more visitors, the local council have 'tidied' it up, replacing the old crumbling walls with safer new ones. The last time I went I felt its energy, its spirit, had almost vanished. Was it dying or was it just quietly moving on, away from the raucous voices and the disrespect?

The same principle can be seen in many of the 'great' sites. Stonehenge has become almost like a creature in a zoo, to be ogled through the fences. The huge temples of Mexico, Egypt and South America are swarmed over by hoards of tourists half-listening to their guides barking out snapshots of information. The pathways that lead up Glastonbury Tor are littered with rubbish; when you reach the top you will most likely meet – not the echoing voice of the wind as it hurls itself around St Michael's chapel, but the beady lens of a camcorder and the shrill tones of pop music.

What is the answer? Find your own sacred sites, your own special places. They lie in every neighbourhood, whether rural, suburban or entirely urban – it just takes a careful eye and an opening of your own energy. And when you do, keep them secret, make them yours. Approach them with reverence and always thank them for their restorative powers. Children find them naturally – so be careful not to blunder into their own private worlds. Visit the old sites but carefully, mindfully. Pick up litter and take it away. Visit in the small hours – at twilight, at sunrise – when coach parties do not visit. Go alone or if you are with others, be silent. Listen, watch, feel. Allow yourself and the place time to get to know each other: sit softly and quietly, just be. Come to learn. Quietly sit and wait for the place to communicate to you. It probably won't happen immediately; it may not happen at all. Shamans spend years building rapport with places. But when and if it does happen, you may find wonderful surprises.

Take time to look at what's around you – the tiny miracles

as well as the large extravaganzas of Nature

SEASONAL ENERGY

It's easier to reconnect with Nature in the summer, when the air is warm and the sun shines. But there is more than one season in the year, and every month, every week, every day, every time of the day is different from the last and the one to come. My great lesson in this came when Monty, the boxer puppy, came into my life. Monty needs two walks a day. Walking with him over our local fields I was amazed at the changing face of Nature. The landscape around where we lived was not dramatic – it was simple farming country. But it changed every day and in every light. Walking and watching put me back in touch with the subtle rhythms of the year. One day a crop would be waving in the fields; the next it would be cut. The plough would furrow the land, turning the earth rich and brown. By evening, the colour would have lightened. Then a soft glow of green would appear – the hint of a fresh crop. Above us the skies would throw a spectacle of clouds, of shifting light, of sunlight and moon-glow.

The key to connecting with the energy of the world around us is not to march, but to meander. And then, every so often, something truly incredible happens. Two hares boxing in the early morning. A cloudscape that looks like floating islands in the reds and golds of the setting sun...

Take every opportunity you can to be out in the open, observing and participating in the world around us.

You don't have to live in the heart of the country to enjoy your changing environment: a city changes too, by season and by the passing hours of the day. The changes may be more subtle but there is still joy in catching them. I remember clearly walking to school as a child. We lived in a suburb and my walk took me along house-lined roads, over a railway bridge and along the edge of a playing field. But every day I saw something new, something wondrous. I was fascinated by tiny plants growing in walls, intrigued by the webs and cocoons built in hedges, moved by the shy wild flowers in odd patches of wasteland. Why lose that child's sense of wonder in the ordinary? When you are out, keep honing your senses to the world around you. Each day you practise this observation you will notice more and more. You'll be amazed at the world going on all around you. Watch the changes as the weeks and seasons change. As you become more sensitive you might even find that your mood and energy are mirrored in some way by the rhythms of the natural world.

THE ENERGY OF THE GARDEN

You can connect with natural energy on a daily basis through a garden. I think everyone needs a 'soul garden', a place, however small, where you can tune in to earth energy on even the tiniest of bases. If you don't have a patch of earth, you might have a balcony or a roof terrace. If you don't even have that you could have your own tiny patch of earth hanging outside your window or place tubs outside your front door. Just having a tiny piece of earth into which to plunge your hands is very healing for your own body energy.

If you have more space, so much the better. A soul garden is just as it says – a garden to soothe the soul and give solace from the maddening world. It doesn't have to be perfect, with regimented flower beds and not a weed in sight. The soul doesn't worry about immaculate rolled lawns. But it does need to be a place in which you can sit, muse, ponder and dream; a place in which you can connect to the earth energy, a place to recharge your energetic

Think about what you need from your soul garden – distill it to its very essence. Is it a heady, romantic garden? Or perhaps a very still, pure, clear spot? Do you want to feel enclosed, surrounded, protected? Or do you crave wide open spaces?

batteries. I love the 'secret' parts of my garden, the hidden places where I can hide away with a book or simply sit, surrounded by the industry of the insects and birds, and the soothing gentle movements of the plants.

When summer and even spring, seem a long way away, nurture your dreams of a soul garden with planning. Sit down and surround yourself with books, gardening magazines and seed catalogues. Browse through old homes and gardens magazines – which pictures draw you? Which elements would you love in your soul garden? It might be a Zen-like corner with beautiful pebbles and a tranquil pool. It could be an untamed wilderness of tall grasses. It could be a hammock with a clear view of trees and sky. What plants are in your garden? Choose the plants you love, not just for their flowers but also for their foliage and their scent. This is an exercise in dreaming. At this point it doesn't matter whether you have acres of space or a tiny roof terrace, a balcony or even a sole window ledge. Think about what you need from your soul garden – distill it to its very essence. Is it a heady, romantic garden? Or perhaps a very still, pure, clear spot? Do you want to feel enclosed, surrounded, protected? Or do you crave wide open spaces? Your image of the ideal soul garden will tell you a lot about yourself and your inner energy needs.

Many of us instinctively turn to images of the kind of garden we had as children – in some way we are craving a return to childhood simplicity, safety, innocence (whether this was or was not a reality for us). If this is the case for you, maybe think about how you can nurture this child-like side. Often we deny ourselves the things we love because we feel we're too 'grown up', too adult and sensible to have them. But why not have a swing in your garden if you want one? Why not grow sunflowers and 'bunny rabbit' snapdragons if you want? Who says a garden needs to be sophisticated? Why feel you should have a 'white' garden because the books say it's fashionable when you adore a chaotic carnival of colours? Why shun petunias and dahlias and French marigolds because they're 'common' if you love them?

So cut out pictures, check seeds and plants in nursery catalogues, ponder gazebos, arches and pergolas. Put them together in your journal or stick them somewhere you can see them – on your fridge door, on your noticeboard. You will also be giving your subconscious the message that this is what you need and crave – as the weeks pass you may find ways arise for your dreams to come true. By putting graphic representations of what we want out there in the world, we are setting an energetic template for our subconscious. Often surprising things happen…

Gardens aren't all dreams of course. There is practical work to be done too.

● If you can, start from seed – there is something magical about buying a packet of seeds and watching them grow into real plants. This is a real exercise in seeing energy manifest itself. Try holding your hands over the germinating seedlings and feel the dynamism of their abundant, fresh energy. Your own energy can help them grow – so direct it to the seeds and seedlings.

● Allow Nature to take her course a little: let seedlings colonize cracks in walls and paths, particularly if they have a sweet scent which is released as you walk over them

● If you have a larger plot, think about giving some of it back to the wilderness. You might plant or preserve a wood (imagine the heady delight of your own bluebell wood); you could allow a meadow to wave its grasses and flowers through the seasons (come summer you could mow pathways to a central circle where you could lie and stare up at the sky, hidden from the world).

● If you have the space, do plant trees. The trees are our planetary lungs; we need them desperately. And you will always have a special relationship with a tree you have planted and tended yourself. Choose, if you can, native species that will feel at home in your space. Take care to prepare the ground properly for them and watch them as they grow.

● Plant a tree to mark a birth, a wedding, arriving at a new home – any excuse will do. And don't be put off planting because you know you will move on: providing you site your trees carefully and considerately, you will be leaving a real gift for the people who come after you – and you can always come back and visit.

● Allow space for the healing scents of herbs. Having fresh herbs at hand's reach makes for wonderful cooking and a free source of home herbal baths (plus creams and shampoos, if you can find time to make them). Even a window-sill can provide a space for a window box or tubs of herbs – and you will catch their scent as you work in the kitchen.

● Plant lavender in boxes outside your bedroom windows and the soothing scent will lull you to sleep. Outside you don't have to limit yourself to herbs in pots and beds. Try planting a chamomile lawn – it smells delicious as you walk over it and you will have a steady supply of fresh chamomile tea to soothe you to sleep. Or edge paths with lavender and chamomile – my dog Monty smells like a herbal pot-pourri when he comes in from the garden!

● Another lovely idea is to make a thyme seat. Fill a wooden or stone trough with well-packed earth right to the top and plant thyme seeds or young plants. Thyme is pretty tough and can cope with being trimmed – and with being sat upon in warm weather. The scent, again, is divine.

CHAPTER TEN

CITIES AND THE WORKPLACE

There is energy in the city as well as the natural world. A different kind of energy, but just as meaningful. If we want to be energyworkers we cannot divide our lives – we should connect with all the various forms of energy we find and work with them rather than focusing only on the 'natural', the 'good' energy. Many people divide their lives into compartments, switching off as they leave home for work, and only switching on again when they leave. Don't fall into the trap of thinking work cannot be energywork.

If you invest your work with a knowledge of vital energy, if you connect fully with its own energy, you will get far more out of your working day.

Similarly it doesn't make sense to ignore the energy of the city, the energy of trains and buses and cars and bustling, frenzied people. Shops have their own energy, the energy of commerce. It will vary as much as the energy between a stone and a leaf. Think of the small neighbourhood store and compare it with the vast hypermarket. Feel the difference in energy. Your corner shop might be full of friendly, bustling local energy or might be suffering from a severe dose of clutter and too much gossip! The supermarket will have a very different energy, generally moving very fast down those long straight aisles. This is why many of us feel uncomfortable in supermarkets. The same happens in malls where there are, once again, those long avenues and sharp corners. Which is why, every time I go into a supermarket or shopping mall, I spend a few moments centring myself and grounding myself. Focus on balancing your chakras. Set up a bubble of protection to shield you from the 'cutting' chi which will be coming at you from all angles. Call on Buffalo to keep you earthed and grounded.

City energy is exhilarating but it can be exhausting. When you live in the city, you become tuned in to its pace. You build your own automatic psychic wall to protect yourself and after a while you learn to blank out the sheer size and enormity of it all. I spent my first 30 years living in cities and so was totally at home in the city. But when I moved out to the countryside I found that, within months, I had lost my 'city-wise' ways. Everything was just too loud, too fast. I had come out of step with the city energy.

The key to dealing with city energy is to become an urban shaman. Take the lessons of the medicine path and apply them to the city.

exercise

SPACE DANCING

This exercise was taught to me by Sue Weston, a wonderful chi kung, tai chi and dance instructor. It's very simple but very useful. It tunes you in to city energy and gives you the space to be able to cope with it.

● Become aware of the people around you as you walk. The aim is not to touch any of them. They will be walking blindly but you must become like a shaman, walking silently through the forest, not making a twig bend or break.

● You are almost 'dancing' your way through the crowds, lithe and nimble you move fluidly and smoothly, sliding through the hoards.

● Anticipate how people will move; look ahead all the time; become aware of the whole space around you.

● Let your vision flit from close distance to middle distance and far distance.

● Send out your energetic feelers to sense where people are. In time you will find you see 'your' path through the crowd and the whole exercise will become supremely effortless.

ENERGY COMMUTING

There are two ways to deal with the horrors of commuting or travelling in cramped conditions on public transport. Firstly you can tune out the whole experience. Simply retreat inside your protective bubble and meditate. You can do this anywhere if you're sitting down, just slump your head forwards everyone will simply think you're dozing.

If you're standing up, sink into the classic chi kung posture: feet shoulder-width apart, knees soft. Imagine a string gently pulling your head up to the ceiling so your neck lengthens and your shoulders relax down. Tuck your chin in and centre yourself by focusing on your solar plexus. Breathe into it feeling yourself relax with every breathe. You can close your eyes or softly blur your gaze. Just concentrate on your breathing.

These techniques are ideal if you are feeling tired or battered. Also, you are far more likely to come across deeply negative people with disturbed energy patterns in the city. Don't feel it's ducking the issue: sometimes closing your energy off is the most sensible course to follow.

If you're feeling energetic and inquisitive, use your commuting time to test out your energy sensing on other people.

If you feel up to it you can practice your aura detection (as explained on page 14) even on a crowded train, but be subtle. Or gently probe into the other person's energy field. Ask permission (silently) and be willing to back off if you feel they do not want to 'meet' you, on an energetic level. But, if they are willing, then see what you can find out. What kind of person are they? How does their energy feel? Is there anything you can learn from them? Anything you can give them in return? If they seem willing, you can give them an 'energy bath'. Pull down vital energy through the crown chakra into your heart chakra and then send it out to their heart chakra, wishing them happiness, health, wealth, whatever you think they need. It's a lovely form of spiritual blessing. This is also something that is good to do if you see someone in pain or trouble. Someone who looks harried or stressed, a mother shouting at her kids or a homeless person begging on the streets. If you can't give financially at least you can give energetically.

CITY MEDICINE

Just as you walked the medicine way in Nature in the last chapter, you can walk mindfully through the city. Keep your senses awake for signs from the energy of the universe. There are birds in the city too – watch the flight of sparrows and blackbird, thrush and wren. You might even see more surprising visitors. I was once in a business meeting high up on the top floor of an office building. It was quite boring and I was almost nodding off, which would have been to my great disadvantage. Suddenly, one of my colleagues pointed out of the window: 'Look, it's a kestrel,' she said with amazement. We all watched the beautiful bird of prey with wonder and came back to our meeting with a renewed sense of purpose and vigour.

Keep an eye out for the lessons of nature within the city. How can a tiny seedling push through the tarmac? Surely only by gently, slowly, surely, insistently making its way, never giving up, never thinking the odds are stacked against it. Now that's a message for modern life, isn't it? Or the plant which will bend and stretch itself to reach the light – we can be flexible too, learning how to move seamlessly, perfectly adapting ourselves to our position. Birds make nests out of incongruous materials – we can look for gold amidst the dross.

There are lessons to be learned from less natural things too. Take notice of the traffic and the cables around you. See connections, ponder artificial forms of energy and how they work in our lives. Notice the buildings around you. Which work well, which fit in with the energy of the city? Which seem out of place, ill-thought, badly designed? Which have good energy, which attract bad energy?

Listen to the rhythm of the train, watch the dance of traffic, follow the lines of telegraph poles and electricity cables

CONSCIOUS MANIFESTATION

Once you start to feel in tune with the energy of the city you can have great fun. One of the rules of energy working is that when you take your conscious attention to something you send energy towards it. Hence you can start to manifest what you desire. This is the basis of all 'magic', all spells and rituals. By paying attention, by focusing your energy, you are affecting the energetic web that surrounds us. Ripples occur and if you have focused your energy effectively something will happen. One way of doing this that is surprisingly efficient and very useful is manifesting parking places. You simply visualize, in perfect detail, where you want to park. See it clearly in your mind's eye, see the area around it, the cars around it. Then visualize a car leaving 'your' space just as you drive up. See your car entering the space and you saying 'Wow, that's great. The perfect space.' If you can really focus, it works. It's a technique I learned from the packet of a little 'parking Buddha' I bought years ago from a joke shop in Boston. But it's far from a joke when you're hunting for parking in the city. I would say the technique works eight times out of ten for me: my concentration isn't always 100% on the task!

Of course, you can use this for pretty well anything else: to summon your bus or train when it's late; to manifest a seat when you're weary; to find a good spot to eat lunch ... whatever.

OFFICE ENERGY

Not everyone works in offices but usually it's the people who do who have the most problems at work! Offices are tricky places, full of all kinds of competing energy. Often they are built on rotten sites and have negative energy from the start. Then they are decorated using materials that emit toxic fumes, which make employees feel sick. Electrical equipment sends out electro-magnetic fields, which interfere with our own energy field, again making us feel off-colour and interfering with our concentration. Few buildings in the West use feng shui or vastu shastra so they have long corridors, angular walls and sharp, pointed desks, which send energy flying out in all directions, making us feel insecure and harassed. Then, as if that were not enough, you're sharing space with all those other people with their worries, hang-ups and concerns. It's one giant energetic melting pot and often very uncomfortable.

But fortunately there are ways to make it better ... let's start by looking at your physical environment and see how its energy can be made more soothing.

THE OFFICE SANCTUARY

Just as you turned your home into a soothing sanctuary full of vibrant healing energy, you need to focus some positive energy in your workplace. The rules are pretty much the same. First of all clear out all the clutter: it's incredibly easy to amass papers and books, journals and notes, and somehow we manage to justify it if it's our work. I used to work with a lovely woman whose desk was a total nightmare. There was so much material stacked on it, under it, around it that you could barely get your legs under the desk and when I tried to find a space to write a message I ended up scribbling on my knee! Needless to say she was always rather flustered and never felt in control. So, don't fall into the clutter trap:

● Have a clear, concise filing system and stick to it. Buy some attractive folders and box files – you might want to cover them with some bright paper or interesting fabric to personalize them. Perhaps you could paint your filing cabinets to add some positive energy to your space.

● Be ruthless about clearing away material you no longer need. Remember you can generally find most information in libraries or on the Internet. Spring-clean your computer files at regular intervals too – it will speed up your computer and be good feng shui for your cyberspace!!

● Open your post over the trash can so you throw away instantly everything you don't need.

● If you can manage it, operate a clear desk policy only have the thing you are actually working on RIGHT NOW on your desk. It makes good energy sense your energy will be focused on the one thing, rather than dissipated amongst several.

● Make time periodically to go through your drawers, filing cabinets and book shelves and get rid of things you no longer need. The clearer your office, the clearer your mind and the easier work will be.

BOOSTING POSITIVE CHI WITH FENG SHUI

Feng shui has plenty to say about office environments. Again we will just look at the easiest, most straightforward advice.

● Your desk should always be positioned diagonally opposite the door, with you facing the door. You need to be able to see everyone who walks in your office immediately. This is the 'power position' and gives you the best energy for control, authority and concentration.

● If you have your back to the door you will, without doubt, feel stressed and uncomfortable. Sitting with your back to the door, whatever your job, can even cause you to be demoted or made redundant. In the manager's office of a large corporation, three supervisors were demoted one after another, within six months of their appointments. They all sat in a desk with their backs facing the door. If for any reason you really can't change your desk position then put up a mirror so you can see people approaching.

● Mirrors can also be used in offices to draw in money-endowing water views (if your office looks out over any kind of water make sure a mirror reflects the view) water is considered to equate with wealth and success. What happens if your desk is immovable and your boss frowns on the idea of mirrors? Slip a mirror into your desk drawer facing the desired direction as a symbolic protection.

● If you are the boss, make sure you don't sit too close to the door of your office, particularly if other workers or secretaries share it with you. If you do you will be treated as an underling and lose respect. Workers in more advantageous positions will become insubordinate.

● If you work for a difficult boss and you have to sit directly in front of, or behind, him or her be sure to place either a crystal paperweight or a bowl of water on your desk. It will deflect any criticism or intolerance. If you can put goldfish in your bowl even better. This really works – I can promise. I tried it with my difficult boss (the one I used to 'love-bomb') and she was much better (although she did once ask why the large crystal appeared to be pointing directly at her!)

● Workers who sit close to the door will tend to leave early and avoid overtime. A mirror positioned to take the worker's attention away from the door will cure the problem.

● If you can, incorporate a fish-tank in your office. A tank with a bubbling aerator is most effective. As previously stated, you should ideally have eight red fish and one black one.

YOUR DESK AS SACRED SPACE

Even if you work in a frenzied environment and can do little about the energy around you, you can have control over your own desk. Make it your own private world, a little sanctuary.

● Keep a bright, functional desk lamp on one side of your desk to help focus your attention. According to feng shui, you can use it to direct energy to a particular part of your working life, depending on where you place it. So, if you want to improve your finances (or maybe get a raise) place it on the far left-hand side of your desk. If work relationships need improving, or you need to 'cast some light' into that area, place it in the top right-hand corner of your desk. Straight ahead of you, it will boost your recognition and fame. In the middle of the right-hand side it will give you a creative edge. In the bottom right-hand side it will make people more helpful towards you. In the bottom right-hand side it will help you if you need to find information or gain knowledge.

● Always try to have fresh flowers on your desk. They stimulate mental activity and cleanse the atmosphere. They are also a lovely reminder of the natural world and have a fresh, cheering energy.

● Your telephone can sit either in the bottom left or right-hand corner of your desk. The right is ideal as it will make people more helpful when you call them. If you are left-handed, keep your address book on your right instead, to gain a similar effect.

● Keep essential reference books on your left-hand side – the knowledge area.

● If your work is creative, try to have a rounded desk. If your work involves figures or is very precise a square desk is better but ideally still with rounded corners.

● Try to use a square briefcase or handbag to make you more inclined to complete projects.

● I always like to have a small candle or tea-light burning while I work. It helps to focus the mind and brings the enlivening energy of fire to your desk. If your co-workers don't mind, you could have an aromatherapy burner, rosemary oil is wonderful for concentration (avoid if you are pregnant or suffer from epilepsy); bergamot is uplifting and the citrus oils are fresh and cheering. If you're feeling very stressed burn lavender. If you can't use a burner, put a couple of drops on a handkerchief or tissue and inhale every so often.

● Crystals are helpful allies on your desk. Cleanse them as on page 127 and dedicate them to help you in your work. Clear quartz will amplify your energy; citrine will help bring in money; turquoise is good for improving communication; garnets boost creativity; amethyst will help you have clear thoughts; obsidian is said to help decision-making.

● If you work in a team, try to have a photograph of you all together in the top right-hand corner of your desk. It will bring you together. You can also put photos of family here, but don't have too many or you will never focus on your work!

● Keep something on your desk which reminds you of your spiritual energy. I have several: a serene Buddha who reminds me to keep calm under stress; an ancient goddess figure who is wonderfully grounding – she has no head (!) reminding me that cerebral energy isn't everything in life! I also have a dancing Shiva figure nudging me to dance lightly through my working life. And a ferocious Balinese demon who guards my desk. Not to mention numerous crystals, candles and affirmations which I stick to my computer. In fact, why not turn your computer into a mini-altar? Lots of people do it automatically and it creates a lovely energy focus on your desk. Of course, it depends on the kind of office in which you work but a few subtle items can always be accommodated.

● Surround yourself with beautiful things. Just because it's an office it doesn't mean everything has to be plastic and generic office equipment. I like to use notebooks which have brightly coloured pages – they lift my energy every time I look at them. Pick a lovely ceramic pot for your pens. Maybe a hand-made willow basket for your in-tray and trash basket?

● Include something from the natural world, ideally something for each element. A candle, a crystal, a bowl of water, a plant. Some plants have the ability to cleanse the atmosphere of electro-magnetic pollution and even toxic fumes. So bring in a spider plant, a peace lily and a sanseviera for clean air.

OFFICE MAGIC

Your attitude and energy will affect the atmosphere of where you work without a shadow of a doubt. If you feel negative and bored with your work, it will be boring. If you consider your workmates dreary, they will drive you mad. But the power to change it lies with you and you alone. If you are stuck in a dead-end job, it can seem natural to simply go through the motions. What a huge waste of your life! Let's look at ways to love the work you do, however humble. The simple key is to invest it with energy: positive, vibrant humming energy.

Let me give you an example. Many years ago I worked as a box office clerk for a large exhibition centre. When the shows were on, I used to sit for eight hours a day in a kiosk, churning out tickets. It would have been the easiest thing in the world to become like most of the clerks: switching off and just working like an automaton. Instead, my friend and I decided we would take a very difficult approach. Instead of dreading the customers we would positively welcome them. We would see just how friendly and helpful we could be. We would aim to connect with each and every customer in a small way while they were buying their ticket. Our second challenge to ourselves was that we would be as speedy and efficient as possible. The change was total. We felt completely energized, immersed in the challenge of being swift AND friendly. The customers seemed to like it too. We had connected with them meaningfully, we had enjoyed an energy exchange – even if only for a few minutes.

You can imbue any task with energy. If you are cleaning a floor, do it mindfully. Turn it into a meditation. Make your actions conscious, turn that floor into a work of art. Bring mindfulness to every action. If you have to deal with people on the phone, try to connect with them via your voice. If you work with numbers, look for patterns. There is truly no form of work that cannot be doused with a liberal sprinkling of positive energy.

I'm a huge believer in oracular systems like the I Ching, the tarot and the runes. And I don't think they should be kept for just fortune-telling or deep spiritual matters. If you have a dilemma at work or want to know how to approach a problem or challenge, consult the oracle. Although it is the most challenging, I find the I Ching the most practical. If you cannot get to grips with the language of the original translation, there are now some excellent modern interpretations I particularly like Sarah Dening's books – see the bibliography.

ENERGETIC MEETINGS

Few of us work in isolation. Before we leave the question of office and work energy let's look at how our energyworking techniques can help our relationships with the people around us. Basically it's a case of applying and adapting the techniques we learned in Part Two. But there are a few other tricks and techniques that can help.

It all comes down to getting along. If you can gain rapport with someone, life becomes a lot easier. We can choose our friends but we generally cannot choose the people with whom we do business. Most difficulties come about because we have different viewpoints, different kinds of energy. If you can bridge the gap, you are well on the way to a more harmonious way of working. Remember, you are the energyworker, so it is your responsibility to get the energy moving smoothly. Don't fall into the blame trap – 'It's his fault'; 'it's not fair', 'well, if she won't make the effort' and so on. Boring isn't it? You have the power to change that. You can influence the other person (in the nicest possible way) by shifting the energy. It's not a case of manipulating them round to your way of thinking but finding the best solution for all of you. Here's how...

1. Make an energetic connection. Follow the technique on page 90 connecting at whichever chakras you need. For most business work it is useful to connect at solar plexus, heart and throat. If your relationship needs grounding then use the base chakra (just watch you don't end up sexually involved!) If you need to connect on an intuitive level, join up at the third eye chakra.

2. If you are in a meeting and want to connect then visualize the bubble of protection extending right around the table. Pull down vital energy through the crown chakra and send it into your heart chakra. Ask everyone else to do the same (best to do this silently, on an energetic level – at least in most workplaces!) Now imagine the energy shooting out from your heart and connecting with everyone else around the table – as if you were all spokes of a giant wheel. Each is connected to each other around the rim; you all join together in the hub. Just like we did on page 58 for linking up at mealtimes. This is a seriously powerful technique and you should feel a real tingling of energy as you connect up. I've known many initially difficult meetings be totally transformed by this. It's also a nice exercise to do if you work in a team – spend a few moments each day connecting with each other in this way.

3. We often meet people with whom we just don't click. If you need to get on, it can be useful to understand their position. For this we can use a simple energy technique – we just step into their shoes. This is also very useful if you are having an argument. Before it develops into something unpleasant, say 'let's take a few minutes break and cool off before we discuss this.' Go somewhere quiet and try this. Sit down and imagine the other person is sitting opposite you. You now put your position to them. Now imagine you are getting up and sitting in their chair – you are becoming them for the moment. If you were them, how would you answer? If you like you can physically put another chair in front of you and physically shift positions (some people find it easier this way). Shift back and forwards, asking questions, gaining insights. Don't leave until you totally understand how the other person feels and why. Now you can go back and have your discussion – use your new-found knowledge wisely.

4. You can also use the above technique if you want to improve your own performance. Simply pick someone you admire and, whenever you are faced with a challenge, go into their shoes and find out how they would face it. In fact you don't even need to model yourself on someone you know or who's alive. All knowledge is held energetically on other planes of existence – some call it the astral plane – and can be summoned at any time. Maybe there's a figure from history you find inspiring – call on their energy and imagine how they would react. Use the strategy of great business people or military commanders; the wisdom of the great philosophers; the humour of the great comedians.

5. Bring playfulness, fun and kindness into the workplace. I've left this until last because I think it's a really important and much forgotten element of working life. Have a kind word for everyone, make an effort to give compliments and praise – as much as possible. Bake a batch of cookies or cakes (with mindfulness, imbuing them with loving energy and any qualities you would like your workmates to enjoy. They could be 'team cookies' or 'creativity cakes' … whatever). You might put initials on them – or a fun symbol for each person. Practise those random acts of kindness – they really are powerful energy shifters. Maybe you could initiate an 'office angel' system. Each person becomes a 'secret angel' to someone else in the office. Every week the angels send their people something small – an encouraging note, an email card, a little posy of flowers. If your person is feeling down, it's up to you to find a secret way of cheering them up. But remember, angels are always anonymous – and don't be tempted to let it get too big (just little notes and cards – not big presents or it ends up as a competition).

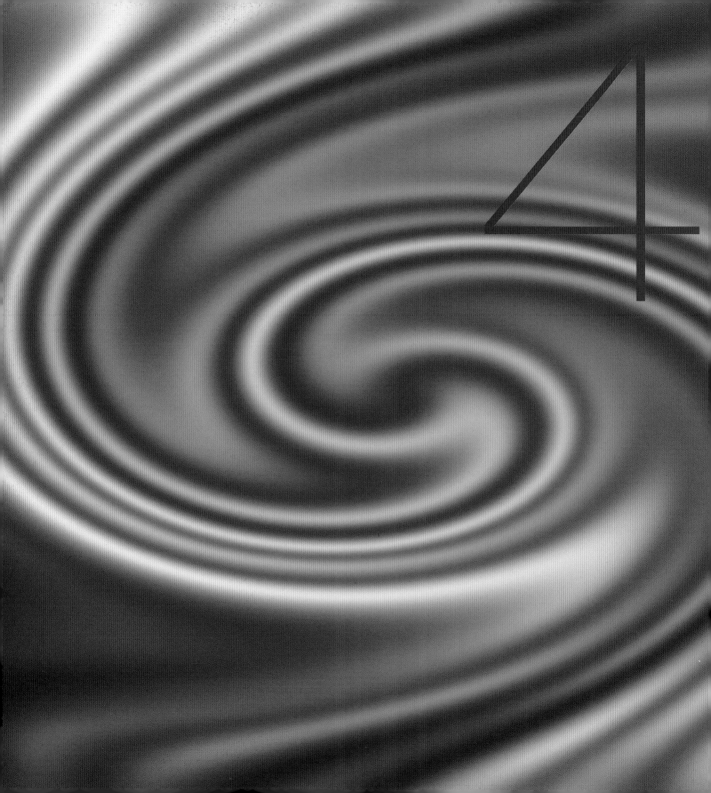

spiritual**energy**

CHAPTER ELEVEN

CONNECTING TO SPIRITUAL ENERGY

Many of us are wary of the word 'spiritual'. Perhaps it reminds us of being dragged to church when we were small, sitting on hard benches listening to boring sermons. Or perhaps it worries us because we are cynical about what we consider 'New Age mumbo jumbo'. Maybe, just maybe, we are scared of what might happen to us if we were to allow ourselves to seek (and maybe find!) the ultimate source of energy. Yet, if you have been following the path outlined in this book, you are already working with spiritual energy. In fact all the divisions are pretty spurious. All energy is spiritual energy. The energy that runs through our bodies, that connects us with other people, that cascades through nature and hums in the city – it is all spiritual. Our bodies and minds are not separate from our souls. They are fused together, each interconnected, each informing the other. It's just how the energy is manifested that differs. Thinking of life and the universe as being energetic in nature is the key to understanding many

Many of us are wary of the word 'spiritual'. Perhaps it reminds us of being dragged to church when we were small, sitting on hard benches listening to boring sermons.

great spiritual truths. When you study the huge variety of religions around the world, all the teachings come down to the same thing. The universe is made up of energy; there is, if you like, one ultimate energy source to which we all belong. Creation can be seen as a huge energy surge which triggered a lightning flash of reactions: pure spiritual energy from the Source started moving down towards material manifestation. Gradually it becomes denser, more capable of creating form. Eventually it becomes solid enough to transform into matter. Our bodies and the physical form of the world around us are born. But, and this is very important, it is still the same energy in essence. We all have within us the divine spark of the original, ultimate energy source. That flame never dies and it can always connect us back to our divine roots. What we will learn in this chapter is how to take more steps towards connecting with the Source. On the way we will learn a lot more about ourselves as well.

My preference for this kind of energyworking is to use the vast wisdom and age-old tradition of the Qabalah. It's something I came across when I was a teenager and have been studying ever since. I love it because it offers a clear map for energyworking, is totally flexible and embraces every form of religious thought and belief. Before we launch into the exercises, it will probably help if I give a brief lowdown.

'See yourself not as a stranger in the universe, not even
diversity in unity, and say I am a Child of Earth, but my

as a separate being apart from it, but as part of that living
Race is from the Starry Heavens.'

W E Butler

THE QABALAH – A MAP OF ENERGY

The Qabalah (also known as the Kaballah, and a host of various spellings) offers a map of creation – from the first intention of 'God' (the original Source) down to the lowliest micro-organism on the earth; from the swirling mass of energy and matter that we are now beginning to understand as the basis of quantum physics to the everyday anxieties and worries that make up our individual psyches. Although the Qabalah is Jewish in origin, it embraces all creeds and religions. And despite the fact that the other great Jewish religious texts (the Old Testament and the Talmud) are so intrinsically male-centred, the Qabalah shows a vision of male and female in perfect balance. Equally it does not shy away from the concept of dark energy. While Qabalistic texts speak of angels and archangels, they also point out demons and arch-demons. Don't be alarmed by the terminology: they are simply ways of pointing to various forms of energy. The Qabalistic world is one of opposites held in balance (just like yin and yang). So perhaps it's not surprising that such a revolutionary system should have stayed underground and relatively unknown to most people for so many years.

The Qabalah can be as simple or complex as you wish. Some people simply use the symbols of the central symbol of the Qabalah, the Tree of Life, as a source of meditation – to help them understand different aspects of themselves or their lives. Others study it in great depth, poring over scholarly texts. Others see it as a true mystical path, offering a direct route to a closer experience of God. And some others use it as part of a magical tradition, to develop power and control over all aspects of themselves and their lives. It is an infinitely flexible system and, as you get to know it better, you will doubtless find your own path.

The Qabalah explains that God created the world by divine speech. As the Bible says: 'God said, "Let there be light", and there was light.' And 'By the word of God the heavens were made; by the breath of his mouth, all their hosts.' However, the Qabalah goes into far greater detail. God used specific sounds, with specific numerical significance, to create the sephiroth – ten spheres that map the energetic path from pure divinity down into the material world. You could say that the true language of the Qabalah is mathematics. Modern commentators also point out that the Qabalah's descriptions of creation can be understood in light of the new physics.

By meditating on the spheres and paths of the Tree of Life it is said that we can gain deep insights into our own natures, into our place in the world and even into the nature of God.

THE TREE OF LIFE

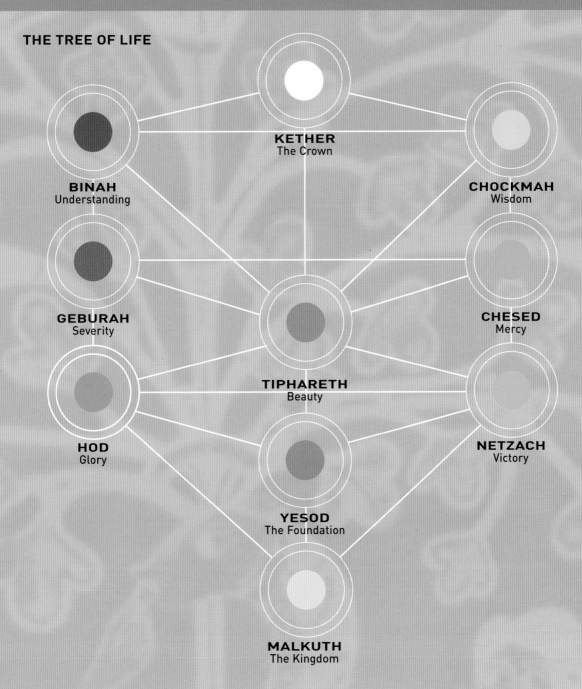

KETHER
The Crown

BINAH
Understanding

CHOCKMAH
Wisdom

GEBURAH
Severity

CHESED
Mercy

TIPHARETH
Beauty

HOD
Glory

NETZACH
Victory

YESOD
The Foundation

MALKUTH
The Kingdom

THE TREE OF LIFE

The Tree of Life lies at the heart of the Qabalah. It offers us a map to the conscious and unconscious, to the world around us and to the many hidden energetic worlds that lie above and below our everyday consciousness. By meditating on the individual spheres, the sephiroth, or travelling the paths from sephirah to sephirah (in a form of guided visualization called pathworking) you can gain an understanding of yourself and start to connect to the various forms of spiritual energy contained within the Tree.

There are vast tomes written on the complex symbolism, meanings and applications of the various spheres on the Tree of Life. These are the basics:

MALKUTH – The Kingdom.
Malkuth corresponds to the body and to the material, outer world, our universe. It is the lowest sephirah, the closest to our everyday life and hence the starting point for all meditative work and journeys on the Tree. It represents the contact between our bodies and the world outside; how we relate to the physical world through our senses. The aim in Malkuth is to see a vision of our Holy Guardian Angel. The main colours of this sephirah are yellow, olive, russet and black flecked with gold. Its symbols include the equal-armed cross, a double cube and the magic circle.

YESOD – The Foundation.
Yesod embodies the subconscious – all the energy we have picked up from our past and carry within us, often repressed, largely unknown. It also holds all our future potential. Yesod is equally linked with our sexual nature and with the moon. The task of Yesod is to balance our selves, to make ourselves whole. Its colours are indigo, violet and very dark purple. Its symbols are perfumes and sandals.

HOD – Glory.
Hod is linked with the mind, the intellect and our will-power. It is the sephirah of communication and its task is to learn true and honest communication, both between the various parts of your self and with others. It is also the sphere linked with magic and spells – with 'mental' energywork. Its colours are violet, purple and orange. Its symbol is the apron.

NETZACH – Victory.

This sephirah is associated with feelings – positive and negative energies such as love and hate, joy and sorrow. The task of Netzach is to learn how to be governed by the 'higher' emotions rather than be at the beck and call of the lower emotions: to cultivate unselfishness, altruism and true feelings of love. Netzach is a beautiful sephirah, concerned also with all manner of creative art – painting, dance, music (whether you participate or observe). Its colours are amber, emerald and olive flecked with gold. Its symbols are the rose, the lamp and the girdle.

TIPHARETH – Beauty.

Tiphareth lies at the centre of the Tree of Life. It is often known as the Christ-centre. Tiphareth represents the centre of the whole person – the Self, the soul – pure self-awareness. The lesson of Tiphareth is to live in harmony, to have a clearly defined sense of self that derives from equal shares of thinking, feeling and sensing. At this point on the Tree the task is to contact and converse with the Guardian Angel (linking yourself with a sense of the eternal, the spiritual). Tiphareth's colours are rose-pink, yellow and rich-salmon pink. Its symbols include the cross, the cube and a truncated pyramid.

GEBURAH – Severity.

Geburah is a tough sephirah of judgment and unmitigated truth. It is linked with personal will and power. When balanced, this brings about strength, order, activity and focused awareness; when unbalanced, it can manifest in manipulation, selfishness, pride, over-ambition and competitiveness. In this sephirah one needs to be totally honest with oneself. Its colours are orange, bright red and scarlet. Its symbols include the pentagon, the sword, the spear and the scourge.

CHESED – Mercy (sometimes known as Love).

This sephirah is concerned with the manifestation of form – not form as we understand matter but rather the 'thought' forms of the mind. The challenge in Chesed is to balance the experience of love – to foster feelings of caring, sensitivity and co-operation without descending into dependence, attachment, the inability to say no and an over-desire to please. The colours of Chesed are violets, purples and blue. Its symbols include the orb, the wand and the sceptre.

DAATH – Knowledge.

Daath is the one sephirah that is not situated on the Tree, it is the mysterious hidden sephirah that lies in the middle of the Abyss, above Tiphareth and below Kether. Many see Daath in a negative light – as representing knowledge without understanding, restriction and dispersion. It is also said to be the prime link to all that is evil and demonic in the world. However, translated into psychological terms, it could be said that the Abyss holds all the unresolved and irrational elements of the psyche and that no-one can cross the Abyss into true spirituality without resolving these aspects.

BINAH – Understanding.

Binah is the first appearance of form on the Tree. Energy is just starting to turn into matter – the primal feminine force. Below Binah lies the 'abyss', the gulf between the actual world below and the potential world above. Binah is known as spiritual awareness and love and the experience of Binah is known as the 'Vision of Sorrow', on one hand an understanding of the full impact of the 'fall' of humanity; on the other a knowledge of the healing power of true grief. The colours of Binah are primarily crimson, black and dark brown. The symbols include the cup or chalice.

CHOCKMAH – Wisdom.

Chockmah signifies spiritual will and purpose, the result of applying spiritual purpose to understanding. The experience of Chockmah is that of seeing God face to face. Chockmah represents the dynamic thrust and drive of spiritual energy – the primal masculine force. The colours of Chockmah are primarily soft blues and greys. The symbols of Chockmah are all phallic symbols – standing stones, the tower, the rod of power.

KETHER – The Crown.

The fount of Creation, where life begins, where there is no distinction between male and female, energy and matter. No-one alive can fully experience this sphere which represents union with God. However, it is said one can glimpse the glory of God through this sephirah. Kether is light, its colours are pure white brilliance and white flecked with gold. The main symbol of Kether is the equal-armed cross, the swastika (which was an esoteric symbol long before the Nazis colonized and abused it).

BUILDING THE INNER TEMPLE

Working with energy on this plane can be a deep, complex affair. It can awaken old, forgotten feelings and cause repressed memories to emerge from our deep unconscious. For this reason, it is sensible to do this work within a safe container, a sacred space. Creating your own personal inner temple is also an important exercise in using your powers of visualization, which need to be strong for this work. And, on a purely practical level, retreating to your own space helps focus the mind.

Your temple is just that – your temple. So create it in a form that pleases you. If you have any religious affiliations then you will probably want to build it on similar lines to where you worship or where you used to worship as a child (if that has pleasant memories).

Why do we go to church or to the mosque, the temple, the synagogue or sacred grove? Because, generally speaking, it is much easier to connect with the spiritual in a place dedicated to the spirit. Although it's not impossible, it's much harder to connect to divine energy when you're surrounded by the detritus (but hopefully not the clutter!) of everyday life. Well, few of us have the space within our homes to dedicate a whole room to our spiritual energy work but that actually doesn't matter at all. For the work we will be doing in this chapter and those that follow, we will be building an inner sanctum, an energetic temple in which to work. In an energetic sense it actually doesn't matter that our temple is in the imagination. Once you have learned how to build it, and use it repeatedly, it will become as real on an energetic level as a physical building made of material bricks and mortar.

Your temple is just that – your temple. So create it in a form that pleases you. If you have any religious affiliations then you will probably want to build it on similar lines to where you worship or where you used to worship as a child (if that has pleasant memories). A temple can be a complex building, a simple room or even a beautiful place in nature. Let's take a moment to think about what a sacred space means for you.

exercise

BUILDING YOUR INNER TEMPLE

1. Sit quietly. Shut your eyes. Become aware of your breathing and bring your focus to your heart chakra. Breathe into this chakra. Become quiet and still.

2. Now bring down energy from the crown chakra. Imagine it streaming in from the universe down into your heart chakra. Just sit for a moment feeling this shiver of vital energy in your body.

3. Now let your mind wander over the idea of a temple. What elements are important for you? Should it be a building or somewhere out in nature? What are its boundaries like? A temple needs to be defined – if it is outdoors think in terms of a ring of trees, perhaps. Or a circle of stones. Perhaps it could be on a small island, or surrounded by a beautiful old wall?

4. Feel your temple. What is the floor like? Is it marble, cool under foot, or warm polished wood? Do your toes curl on woodland moss or feel sun-kissed sand? What are the walls made of? Are there windows? What is the temperature in your space?

5. What decoration does your temple have? Are there tapestries, stained glass windows, sacred symbols or is it plain?

6. Imagine the altar. How do you see it? Is it beautifully carved from wood or a rough-hewn stone? What items will you have on it? Traditionally one would have something to represent each element. Hence a candle for fire, incense for air, salt or bread for earth and water or wine for water. How does the incense smell? Feel the salt run through your fingers; break off a piece of the bread. Lift the cup (what kind of cup?) to your nose and smell the wine or sweet freshness of the water.

7. What would you wear in your temple? Feel the fabric (if indeed you are wearing clothes)against your body. Look at your feet.

8. Every temple has a guardian, be it an angel, a nature spirit or a power animal. What would be the guardian of your temple? Do you already have a connection with it? If not, could you make one?

If you find this exercise difficult, let me give you a blueprint for a temple which works very effectively for me.

The Temple of Malkuth

This temple already has a lot of power and comfort invested in it as it is one of the temples on the Tree of Life. Malkuth is the sphere of energy that is most solid or material – it is the 'earth' temple. I have found this a wonderful temple with which to work: it is based on one described by Dolores Ashcroft-Nowicki (see bibliography) and is similar to the masonic Solomon's temple.

The wall in front of you has three heavy oak doors, with no handle or locks. In front of the doors are two pillars which stretch from the floor up to the ceiling. The one on the left (as you look at it) is made of gleaming black ebony. The one on the right shines softly silver.

The temple is square; its floor made of black and white tiles. In the middle of the temple stands an altar, two hand-crafted cubes (one on top of the other) of black wood, well-polished by loving hands. Over it lies a linen cloth and on top of that is a beautiful bowl made of electric-blue crystal. Inside the bowl a light steadily burns. Next to it sits a loaf of freshly baked bread and a bronze cup containing a rich, fruity red wine. Above the altar, hanging down from the ceiling, is a bronze censor in which burns a light, fragrant incense.

The wall in front of you has three heavy oak doors, with no handle or locks. In front of the doors are two pillars which stretch from the floor up to the ceiling. The one on the left (as you look at it) is made of gleaming black ebony. The one on the right shines softly silver.

The other three walls all have stained glass windows which send a soft, bejewelled light into the temple. On the window behind you there is an Eagle, soaring into the sky. In the right-hand window is a winged Lion, surrounded by flames. In the left-hand window is a winged Bull, stamping on the earth. Note how similar these are to the Native American power animals – if you wish you could substitute Bear for Lion and Buffalo for Bull.

The guardian of the Temple of Malkuth is the archangel Sandalphon. Imagine him as a tall young man with eyes full of wisdom and compassion, tinged with sadness (after all he is the angel of Earth and feels keenly how we hurt our Mother Earth). He wears a long robe which shimmers with the hues of autumn – russet red, gold, earthy brown, soft green.

● Spend time just being in this temple. Look around and ponder the meaning of the symbols in this temple. Meditate on them and see if you find any illumination.

● 'Talk' to Sandalphon – with deep respect. Ask for his teaching. Listen in silence.

● Clean the temple. Imagine making it sparkling clean – get down on your knees and scrub! Replace the bread and wine every day. Yes, it's metaphorical spring-cleaning but no less real for that.

● Spend time sitting in front of the altar, meditating by gazing at the living flame.

● Remember this is a supremely safe place. If ever you feel anxious or worried you can always come here to retreat. Ask Sandalphon for help in transforming your negative feelings. As you leave imagine any negative energy being purified by the flame on the altar.

JOURNEYING

Once you have built your temple, you can use it as the base for a series of explorations into the energetic worlds that surround us. Many mystical and magical traditions use a technique involving creative visualization to move in energetic worlds that exist outside our material everyday world. The purpose of such journeying is not just for curiosity but to learn. There are several ways of doing this:

Freeform Journeying:

This is very much a case of 'let's go and see what happens.' It's often used in shamanic traditions where there are believed to be two energy worlds outside our own: the lower realm and the upper realm. You can journey to either, starting off in your temple and then either descending or ascending. A door might open, with steps leading down (to the lower realm) or up (to the upper realm). Many people use a visualization of a hollow tree – going down through its roots to the lower realm and climbing up to the top (like Jack in the Beanstalk – a classic 'journey') for the upper world.

It can be useful to take a guardian with you, because you may come across some strange, and possibly even frightening, people or creatures. Remember these are 'your' creatures and probably need dealing with. So ask them what their purpose is, what you need to do. Your guardian can act as a protector, a psychic bodyguard, so the experience is not too scary. When you come back from your journeying make sure you ground yourself well. Stamp your feet, have a drink and something to eat. Write down your experiences and insights.

Guided Journeying:

I actually think it helps (particularly for beginners) to have some kind of blueprint for your journey. The most effective tools for this kind of journeying are the tarot cards or the runes. In the Qabalistic tradition, you would gradually ascend the Tree of Life, experiencing each sephirah and the paths between them (each of which is governed by a tarot card – see the illustration on page 165). A very useful exercise is to spend time meditating on each of the sephirah. Look back at the correspondences given for each sephirah. Think how it applies to you. Ponder the symbols – what do they mean to you? Each sephirah acts as a mirror of the soul, a connection to the various forms of spiritual energy.

Here are some thoughts to get you started on the first two sephiroth.

● **MALKUTH:**

Think about the elements that constitute our Earth: water, earth, air and fire. Imagine these forces in their natural states. Feel their energy and power. Think about how we abuse the Earth, how we pollute the elements with our waste. Find a connection with our Mother, Earth. Think about what it means to live on this Earth, to be its guardians. Are we honouring that trust?

● **YESOD:**

Think about the people in your life – from those you know now to those with whom you shared your past – right back to your childhood. Allow all your old thoughts and dreams to rise to the surface; your old hopes and disappointments, your old faults and bad habits. Think back to your sexual relationships – were they a good, healthy exchange of energy or were they manipulative or harmful?

exercise

USING THE TAROT OR RUNES

As I've already mentioned, you can use the tarot cards or rune stones as a doorway to energy-journeying. I find the tarot cards easiest and use the Rider Waite pack.

1. First pick out a card. You can either choose to work just from the Major Arcana or the whole pack. You may know the card with which you wish to work – or you may decide to allow the energy of fate to take a hand and just pluck one from the pack.

2. Sit quietly somewhere where you will not be disturbed. If you like, light a candle and draw a bubble of protection around you. Focus on your breathing and centre yourself by breathing into your solar plexus chakra.

3. Now construct your inner temple. Imagine its every detail and then walk into it, feeling your feet on its floor.

4. Imagine a curtain before you – in the Malkuth temple it would hang over the middle door. It could, however, hang from two trees or rocks – or just appear in thin air (energetic worlds do not need to follow the same rules as the physical one!)

5. As you gaze at the curtain an image appears on it of your tarot card, as if on a tapestry. See the card in all its detail.

6. As you walk closer to the curtain you notice that the image is alive and moving. The edges seem to blur and blend into the world outside.

7. Walk into the curtain and feel yourself step into the world of the tarot card. Look at the scene around you. What happens next? Some cards invite you to walk further into their landscape. Some seem to demand that you meet and converse with the beings depicted.

8. Hopefully you will gain some important insights or learn some new knowledge. When you feel you are ready, turn around and walk back. The curtain will appear again and you should walk through it (don't forget to thank any beings with whom you have spoken).

9. You will walk back into your temple. The curtain will fade away. Spend some time quietly thinking about your experience. You may want to discuss it with Sandalphon or your guardian. Give thanks at the altar before you go.

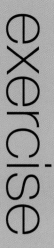

TONING THE NAMES OF GOD

This exercise has obvious links with the chakra balancing exercises we have already practised. This time you will be toning some of the Qabalistic names of God or spiritual energy. It is a very powerful exercise which will help you connect to spiritual energy in a balanced way. It is also supremely protective. If ever you feel uneasy, use this technique to feel yourself connected with the ultimate Source of energy, light and love.

1. Stand facing East and close your eyes. Breathe quietly and deeply, centring yourself as always.

2. Imagine that there is a sphere of pure brilliant white light just above your head. A beam of gleaming white light shoots down from this sphere into your head. As you do this tone the word EHEIEH (pronouned Eh-hay-yay) slowly several times. Imagine the name vibrating over your head – this is your own spiritual energy being brought down from the universal source of spirit.

3. Now the beam of light descends into your throat area where it spreads out to become a shining sphere of gleaming white. The name here is JEHOVAH ELOHIM (Ye-ho-vah El-oh-heem). Intone it into the sphere so you feel the whole area become activated with vital energy.

4. Now the light shoots down to your solar plexus and transforms into a sphere, again of shining white. Say the name JEHOVAH ALOAH VA DAATH (Ye-ho-vah El-oh-vay Da-art) into this sphere. You will feel a warmth spreading out over the area.

5. The light now descends to the area of your genitals. Tone the name SHADDAI EL CHAI (Sha-dee El Key) into this sphere. The syllable 'key' is guttural, more like the 'ch' in loch. If you find your attention wandering, gently bring it back to the name and the gleaming sphere.

6. Finally, the light shoots down through your thighs and calves to your feet where it forms a large sphere from the ankles reaching down into the earth. Imagine you are rooted firmly in this sphere. Tone the name ADONAI HA ARETZ (A-don-ee Ha A-retz).

7. Now visualize the entire shaft of brilliant silvery light which reaches from the crown of your head to the soles of your feet. It is studded with five shimmering spheres which glitter like diamonds. You have activated the middle pillar of the Tree of Life within your body – the effects will remain with you always. Try to repeat this as often as possible – it links you to a balanced form of spiritual energy in a safe, effective way.

As you become accustomed to this exercise you can add some fine-tuning. Each sphere is linked with an element and colour – you can replace the shining white with the various colours – and meditate on the elements assigned to each sphere, figuring out why each belongs where it does.

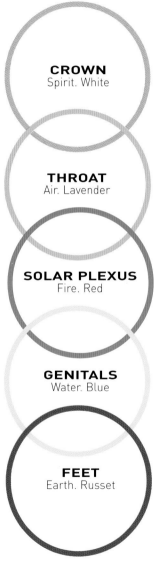

CROWN
Spirit. White

THROAT
Air. Lavender

SOLAR PLEXUS
Fire. Red

GENITALS
Water. Blue

FEET
Earth. Russet

BRINGING SPIRITUAL ENERGY INTO YOUR CELLS

This last exercise brings spiritual energy into your body to be used in whatever way you need. You can focus purely on its spiritual quality, or direct it for physical or emotional healing.

1. Send your attention up to the crown sphere. Imagine it revolving, absorbing spiritual energy from the higher planes and transforming it so you can use it here on the lower plane.

2. Then visualize (and feel) this energy flowing like a stream down and through the left hand side of your head, neck, body, and the left leg. Exhale slowly as it descends.

3. As you slowly inhale, visualize the current passing from the sole of the left foot to the sole of the right foot and gradually ascending the right-hand side of the body. From the head it returns again to the crown. Continue this circulation of energy for several breaths.

4. Now visualize the flow of spiritual energy streaming from the crown down the front of the face, chest, and down to the feet where it turns under the soles of the feet and goes up the back to the crown again. Exhale as it goes down the front; inhale as it comes up the back. Continue for several breaths until it is firmly established.

5. Finally, focus your attention on the base, earth sphere. This is the receptacle of all the energy of the other spheres. Now imagine this power and energy being drawn up through the body through all the other central spheres to the crown. It shoots up the body and erupts through the crown like a fountain of light and energy. The fountain showers down around your body, outlining the aura. Inhale as the energy ascends the body, exhale as it showers down.

6. Imagine your whole body surrounded by bright spiritual energy. You realize that every cell of your body is being suffused by this divine energy. This is the time to direct the energy, should you so wish.

This is not a quick path – you cannot 'learn' spiritual energy in a week, a month or even a decade. It is a lifelong task, one which should be approached with dedication and humility, with a willing and open heart. I am very aware that one chapter is far too short to come to grips with such vast ideas. But I felt it was worthwhile to at least introduce them. You now have at your disposal all the basic tools for a lifetime's journey of discovery. Anyhow, curious souls will always find their own path.

exercise

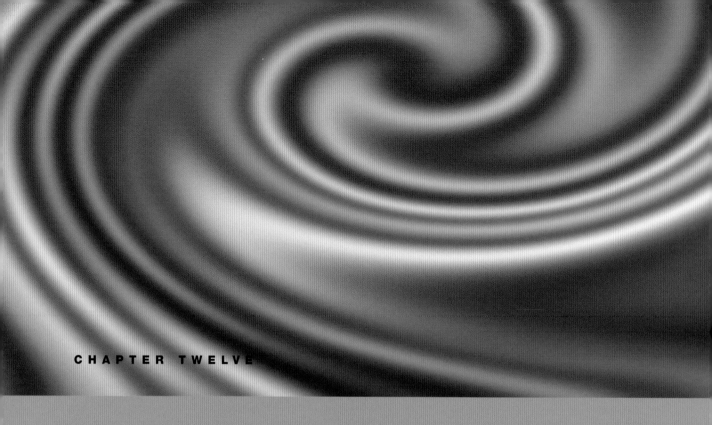

CHAPTER TWELVE

HONOURING DARK ENERGY

Strive for the light, always the light. We are living in a society that has become obsessed with the bright, with the light, with the positive. Within this gleaming bright world there is no room for shadow, for penumbra, twilight, darkness. We have turned our backs on the harsher, more difficult side of life – we just don't want to know.

New Age consciousness has promoted a world of permanent sunshine, of bright colours, rainbows, smiles and hugs. Its buzzwords are love, light, joy, peace, beauty. Its key concepts are affirmations, angels and positive thought. We are taught that we can never afford the luxury of a negative thought', let alone negative emotions or actions. The message is that our lives should be permanently sunny, happy and joyous; all our relationships loving; all our spirits coursing towards the light. We are expected to be super-people, always up, always cheerful, always bright.

By striving for perfection, for the ideal life, we are setting ourselves up for misery and failure. No-one can live perpetually in the bright sunshine. Life is made up of darkness as well as light.

Is this natural? Is it realistic? Of course not. Virtually all of us have times when we feel down, depressed, negative. Times when we feel consumed with less than ideal emotions: anger, hate, jealousy, self-pity. If we were to believe some of the self-help gurus, we would seek to expunge such emotions immediately, drowning them in positive affirmations and self-talk. But is this missing the message? Do we miss the subtlety of the moon's shadows by always craving the clear illumination of the sun? By striving for perfection, for the ideal life, we are setting ourselves up for misery and failure. No-one can live perpetually in the bright sunshine. Life is made up of darkness as well as light. Our emotions too run into the shadows: fear, guilt, depression, anger. We cannot put a veneer over these emotions and simply hope they will simply go away. In fact, the more we disown these emotions, the more harm they will do. It's like finding a patch of nasty damp in your house. You could face it square-on and root out the cause or you could simply paper it over and forget about it. We all know what happens if you go the latter route: all looks fine for a while but eventually the damp breaks out again, far worse than before.

Do we do ourselves a disfavour by ignoring the dark

and seeking always the light?

We only have to look at nature to see that there exists cruelty, darkness, death. There are times of growth, times of decay. Sometimes day and light and the upward surge of life hold sway; sometimes we are in the grip of night and dark and the death-hush lies over the earth. We are splitting from an essential truth if we seek to live always in the light. After all, in order to have a peak, a mountain, you must have a trough, a valley. How can we truly know happiness if we have never experienced sadness and gloom?

By denying the dark we also lose the chance for genuine self-understanding and growth. There are many lessons to learn amidst the shadows, much wisdom in the gloom. We can and should sacrifice the idea of perfection because none of us is perfect. We all contain within us both good and evil, light and shade. When we turn and face our darkness, our demons of the night, we may find revelations beyond our wildest dreams. For there is dark energy too...
The ancients knew this and knew it well. In the Qabalah, the Tree of Life has a shadow image, a dark reflection. On it are all the sins and temptations known, the arch-demons of the soul. The Qabalists realized that you cannot only see the bright side of life, you have to accept the dark as well. To ignore the dark, to push it aside, is to give it power over you. In many cultures the gods and goddesses were not just pure and good but complex creations with as many differing moods and attributes as us humans. Many initiation ceremonies demanded that the initiate descend into the bowels of the earth or go deep into the forest or out onto the untamed sea to face his or her demons, to conquer fear, to embrace the dark and come out again, transformed, into the light.

I am not saying that affirmations and positive thought are bad things. They are in fact incredibly useful and worthwhile, particularly if you are the kind of person who constantly dwells on the negative. They are also valuable lessons in the first stages of energyworking. But once you have reached a certain level of skill in this work you no longer need to put a gloss on life. You are ready to face the darker side. Our first task is to face the shadow...

SEEKING OUR SHADOW

As children we were scared of the dark, of ghosts and ghouls, demons and monsters. When I was small I had nightmares of a black cat-like creature which stalked me relentlessly throughout my childhood, through my teens and into adulthood. For years I sought to exorcise it, to avoid it, to ignore it and hope it would forget me and go away. It wasn't until I started to study Jungian psychology and become fascinated with art therapy that I dared face 'my' beast. For, rest assured, every dark creature of the night, every ignoble thought and deed, is yours and yours alone. And in them lies a chance for huge reward and growth.

My black beast turned out to be something quite wonderful – my own repressed animal self, my wild feminine energy, my sensuality, my inner 'wild woman'. She appeared as I painted: first a terrifying monster that I barely dared look at, gradually transforming into a powerful Sekhmet, Egyptian lion goddess; a sinuous dancer; a delicious strumpet. I realized that here was a huge part of myself that I had always denied, always repressed. She contained my shadow material, my dark energy, which craved release. In Jungian psychology, the shadow is the part of us that contains our secrets, all the forbidden feelings and ways of behaviour that lie hidden from our consciousness. The shadow comes most strongly to us in our dreams, as that frightening 'other' – usually the same sex as ourselves. The harlot, the vicious murderer, the cunning thief, the loud-mouthed zealot, the overbearing teacher, the pathetic wimp, the down-and-out, the whining child. The shadow carries everything that we push aside in waking, conscious life: all those qualities that do not fit with our ideal image of ourselves, everything that makes us embarrassed, shameful, small.

The shadow is thus full of hate, rage, jealousy, shame, laziness, aggression, greed, lust, untrammeled sexuality.

If we do not pay attention to these dark energies they take on a life of their own; they fester in our unconscious; they plague us in dreams, in unbidden fantasies and urges. Sometimes they surface dangerously as when we 'lose it' and hit out in a sudden uncharacteristic bout of fury, or we get blind drunk and wake up next to a stranger, feeling stunned and horrified that we just 'weren't ourselves' last night. We weren't our selves – we were our shadow.

However, we shouldn't seek to destroy the shadow, but to integrate it into our conscious lives, so its immense hidden energy can be used for our own good. Let's look at how to do this.

exercise

SHADOW-WORKING

● Make a list of the people who annoy you most, who really irritate you. They can be close family, passing acquaintances, people on television, a huge celebrity or the woman at the corner shop. Why do they annoy you so much? Which qualities are particularly irritating? Write down everything you hate about them. Take it further and think if there are any groups of people you really can't stand; that you find frightening or repulsive or unpleasant. Be brutally honest with yourself. Don't lie to yourself – even if your thoughts seem atrocious. You're looking for those qualities you just can't stand in other people. 'He's so arrogant,' you might say or 'I hate the way she flaunts her body'. We project our shadows onto other people so, ten to one, the qualities you hate in someone else will be exactly what is hidden in your own shadow. Think about it – is the hated quality something you possess in yourself, or that lies hidden within you?

● Take notes of your dreams. Keep a dream journal and watch out for the shadow figures in your dreams. The shadow will always be the one who enacts the dark and the forbidden: the thief, the murderer, the rapist, the sadist, the prostitute, the beast.

When you have found some of your shadow energy, your shadow characters, you can start working with them. Try these ways to unleash and integrate shadow material:

● Use the 'other chair' technique. Sit on one chair and imagine your shadow character (from a dream or a person you dislike) on the other. Start up a dialogue. Ask them why they behave the way they do. What do they dislike about you? What do they want to say? What do you want to say to them? Try taping your 'conversation' so you can replay it later – you may find some big surprises.

● Paint your shadow. This can be very powerful so don't be surprised if unexpected emotions emerge. Use whatever materials you like. I found it therapeutic to paint large – pinning a huge sheet of paper on the wall and using cheap poster paints. You might choose to work small with gouache, or doodle with felt pens. Sometimes the picture just seems to take you over and paint itself. You may find it helpful to paint in candlelight or the dark (the shadow seems to emerge more readily than in the bright light of day). If you find it hard, you may want to close your eyes or paint with your non-dominant hand. Don't censor yourself – just paint freely. Once you have finished try talking to your painting. Take the image and use the other chair technique or write to it, as outlined below.

● Write to your shadow figure. Just free-associate and see what emerges. It could be a dialogue; it could be a narrative; it could be a poem or a play. Maybe the shadow figure itself wants to write – what would it say? How would it express itself?

Be constantly on the watch for shadow material. Listen to your dreams and keep the dialogue going. Watch out for those irritating people and analyze why they are so grating on your nerves. Who do you envy? Who envies you? Why? What would you love to be able to say, but feel you can't? What would you say if you had the chance? What would be the consequence? If you could change your life in any way, how would you change it? What are your deepest desires, your most wild, wanton fantasies? And what desires are you hiding when you over-eat, drink to excess, take drugs or over-work? What parts of your life are you denying? These are the thoughts we dare not think because we fear that, were we to imagine the unimaginable, we would have to play out our fantasies. But that's not the case. Often all our psyche needs is to air the possibilities, to find small, safe ways to unleash our shadow. Our inner wild woman might cherish a swim in the sea or half an hour lying on her back staring up at the clouds. Our inner warrior might need to unleash some energy in an aerobics class or kick-boxing or screaming out loud in a place where no-one can hear. Simple things might fit the bill very well. If you're not sure, ask your shadow.

You need to face the dark energy, to plumb the depths: only then can you truly scale the heights

PLUMBING THE DEPTHS

Sometimes we find ourselves in very unpleasant places. Life overwhelms us, we feel as if we just cannot carry on, we are consumed by grief, depression, anxiety or fear. Many people say you just have to pull yourself together. I'm not so sure. I think life is a quest for meaning rather than blind happiness. Happiness is a child's pursuit and as we grow up we need more. We start searching for meaning, and meaning can be found in the darkest of places. Most of our lives are spent running away from confrontation, from having to think or face reality. We avoid ourselves in myriad ways – through overwork, alcohol, drugs, watching television, going out. We are scared of standing alone, quiet, naked before the vastness of the universe. We quail before infinity. We are terrified of looking at ourselves honestly and facing what gazes back at us. Those who sink into darkness and gloom are perhaps just a little more honest – they peer through the curtains of illusion. They see the depths but just cannot reach out again.

Another mistake we make is to blame the past. We blame things that happened years ago for our present misery. Yes, terrible things can have happened in the past and they can certainly affect us in the present. But, if we want to grow we have to take responsibility for ourselves, here and now. We have to let go of the past and figure out what we need to do now to move forwards. The key is to learn how to forgive ourselves, to resist apportioning blame, to take responsibility for our own lives, not give it up to those bogeymen of the past.

One way of doing this is to grapple with our own dark energy: to follow the path of the old initiates and make a descent into the underworld. It is to face the worst that could possibly happen – the stripping of everything we hold dear. Then, when we stand alone, forlorn and without all our worldly trappings, we realize we have an essential Self which transcends all the glitter and ego. That is a deeply comforting and empowering experience.

Many people who suffer grief or depression naturally follow a descent. They simply cut off from the world for a time. As long as such a descent is not allowed to continue on for too long, I think this can be a helpful, healing process. Sometimes the psyche just needs to shut down, to rest, to renew. Other people find such a descent can become necessary when they are going through a transitional phase of their lives. It is a process that can challenge many of our assumptions. It is a meeting with dark energy that can be deeply transforming and, paradoxically, end up giving us more bright, vital energy than you can imagine.

THE DESCENT OF INNANA

For this descent I use the myth of Inanna. Inanna was a Sumerian goddess from around the third millennium BC. Sumeria lay in what is now modern-day Iraq, but then it was not a desert but one immense garden – full of vineyards, cornfields, orchards of date palms, olive and fruit trees, pasturelands for cattle, sheep and goats. Inanna seems to have descended from the Bird and Snake goddesses of Neolithic times. She was a complex goddess of life, love and death. She seems more human than many goddesses, more understandable somehow, because her trials and tribulations are those of everyone. She starts out young, reckless, fearless, exulting in her power. She has power in her role as Queen. She learns wisdom and becomes a good ruler. She honours and respects her body and her emerging sexuality. She is very frank about her needs and prepares herself for love and takes a lover,

She was a complex goddess of life, love and death. She seems more human than many goddesses, more understandable somehow, because her trials and tribulations are those of everyone.

Dumuzi, and then weds him and makes him King. She has children and brings them up in love – she loves them and they love her. Then, almost unexpectedly, she decides to take on the most difficult task of all – to descend to the underworld, to transform her own soul. She goes down to the underworld where her sister (and shadow) Ereshkigal, rules.

As she descends into her sister's realm she is stripped of everything until she stands before Ereshkigal naked.

When she meets Ereshkigal she is killed with a glance, beaten and hung from a meat-hook like a slab of meat. She stays there for three days and putrifies. Meanwhile, her priestess Ninshubar, who has been warned to fetch help if she doesn't return, asks three gods for help. The first two refuse but the third agrees and makes creatures from the dirt under his fingernails. These, not being made of flesh and blood, can slip into the underworld and are instructed to go and sympathize with Ereshkigal who is suffering birth pains. She appreciates their concern and offers them first food and drink, which they have been warned to refuse. She then asks them what they would have as a reward and they ask for the body hanging on the hook. Ereshkigal gives them Inanna and they revive her body. She is now free to leave the underworld but she is accompanied by demons who demand she fulfill the decree of the underworld – that the body count must remain the same so, if she leaves, she must send someone else in her place. They suggest Ninshubar but Inanna says no, she has been good and faithful; they cannot have her. Then they come across Inanna's two sons but she cannot bear to lose them. Finally they come to her husband Dumuzi who is sitting on her throne in splendour, happily carrying on the business of being a King without Inanna. He is 'dressed in noble garments ... sitting on a lofty throne'. Inanna is furious and she 'fastened the eye of death, spoke the word against him, the word of wrath.' It is now her, not her sister, who is the underworld, death-dealing goddess – she has integrated Ereshkigal's powers. She offers the demons Dumuzi. Dumuzi is horrified and tries everything he can to escape his fate. He slips away from the demons and hides. They track down his sister Geshtinanna and torture her to

Each gate could be seen as one of the chakras, so giving up each garment corresponds with opening, or laying bare, each centre.

reveal where he is, but she does not tell. They find him anyhow and drag him away but he pleads with Inanna for mercy. Geshtinanna offers to go in his stead and Inanna agrees that they can divide the time, each taking half the year. Dumuzi is taken away.

This is a complex myth and all its elements are well worthy of meditation. However, for now we will focus just on the descent. As Inanna descends, she reaches seven gates and at each she takes off a piece of jewellery or clothing. Each gate could be seen as one of the chakras, so giving up each garment corresponds with opening, or laying bare, each centre. To my mind, they can be seen as the trappings of our egos, our personas, the masks we wear to meet society, to hide from our primal fears and dodge our true selves. This ritual allows us to strip ourselves bare and reveal our inner being.

exercise

1. Find a place and time when you will not be disturbed. Ideally it should be dark and warm. Lie down on the floor (make yourself comfortable with a rug and pillow) and spend a few minutes centring yourself, focusing on your breathing and connecting to your solar plexus.

2. Visualize yourself as Inanna, the great Queen of Sumer. You sit on your wondrous throne, enjoying power and prestige. You are wealthy beyond compare – your wish is your command. Beside you sits your husband Dumuzi, you have a wonderful marriage and enjoy a blissfully good sexual relationship. Your children are good and bright and beautiful. You have good friends and an interesting social and intellectual life. You want for nothing.

3. Yet something is missing. You feel a need to visit your dark sister Erishkegal who lives in the gloom of the underworld. You kiss your family good-bye and tell only your dearest friend where you are going. Then, dressed in your best clothes and finest jewellery you set off on your perilous journey.

4. You walk across fields of swaying corn, dotted with poppies and cornflowers. Birds are singing and the sun shines brightly. The whole world seems beautiful and part of you yearns to sit and picnic, then to return home. But you see ahead of you a range of mountains, and you know that your quest leads you there.

5. You come to a fast-flowing stream over which lie stepping stones, leading to a dark cave. As you walk into the shadow of the rocks, you feel a chill run over your body but you continue bravely. You step into the cave and it seems as though all the light and warmth of the world has vanished.

6. A small light glimmers and you pick up a tiny lantern. At the back of the cave lies a small passageway and you squeeze yourself through this and along a narrow corridor. The path steps steeply downwards and you feel as if you are going into the bowels of the earth.

7. Suddenly a large figure looms before you. It is Neti, the Chief Gatekeeper of the Underworld. Behind him lies the first gate that leads to Erishkegal's realm. 'Welcome Inanna, Queen of Heaven and Earth,' says Neti, 'if you would come to the Dark Kingdom you must shed your fine crown.' You take off the crown and with it all your lofty aspirations, your pretentions to spirituality, your feeling of being better than other people. You drop that 'holier than thou' aspect and walk through the gate with Neti.

8. On you walk, down and down, until you reach another huge gate. Neti asks you if you want to continue and, when you say yes, he asks for your earrings. With these you have to give up the pride you feel over your special abilities, the sense of being different. You take off the earrings and become quite ordinary.

9. Down the path goes and then before you is another gate. This time Neti asks for your necklace and you give it up, along with your power of speech, your clever words, witty repartee, your bright conversation. You leave behind your intellect, your quick mind, your smart thoughts. Neti allows you to go on through, further into the dark and deep.

10. The next gate looms and here you are asked to give up the beautiful breast plate that covers your heart. Here you leave behind all affairs of the heart, all relationships, all emotional attachments, all feelings of love and affection. Feeling quite cold and alone now you walk through.

11. At the next gate you come to Neti asks for the thick belt that winds around your solar plexus. He takes with it your power and will, your intentions and desires. All the striving and strategies fall away.

12. You are now getting deep into the bowels of the earth and the sixth gate comes into view through the darkness. Neti smiles grimly and you hand him the shimmering skirt which has kept your lower body covered. With it he takes your sexuality and your sensuality. He takes too your reproductive powers, your children and potential children, your heirs and your genetic link to the future.

exercise

exercise

13. Now it is becoming very cold. You shiver as you reach the seventh and final gate. Neti seems almost pitying as he asks if you want to continue. You grimly nod and hand over your sandals. With them he takes your home, your place on the earth, your centre, your security. You are left naked and vulnerable.

14. You are ushered into the presence of your dread sister, Ereshkegal, the dark goddess of the underworld. She is huge and frightening and you feel very small in front of her. Take a while to recognize the feelings that come up. How does it feel to stand naked, with nothing? What do you recognize in Ereshkegal? What does she make you face? Can you see that you two are parts of one whole?

15. You step forward and Ereshkigal strikes you dead. She picks up your body and hangs it on a meat-hook. You hang there and recognize that you could remain here, slowly disintegrating, rotting. The dross in you is dying, is being swept away. But the essential 'you' still remains. What is this 'you'? What does it consist of? What is your divine spark? What is your true self? Take some time to discover how it feels to have nothing left of ordinary reality.

16. Slowly you become aware that an exchange is being made. You are being ransomed and will return to life. Before this happens spend some time thinking about how you would like to return; what qualities you would like to take with you; what you would like to leave behind. Remember this is a powerful chance to shed anything you don't want or need any more; to abandon old forms of behaviour that no longer serve you.

17. Ereshkigal gently lifts you from the hook and holds you to her breast. You feel her now as warm and sisterly, not an avenging death goddess. She breathes new life into you and you feel fresh, like a new-born baby. You thank her for the lessons you have learned and you hug, as equals. You promise you won't ignore her but will integrate her dark energy into your life. She hands you a simple white linen dress and a pair of sandals.

18. Slowly you retrace your steps through the seven gates. At each one Neti offers you your own adornments. Do you want them? Do you want to re-evaluate them? Think carefully before you take them back or discard them totally. You may wish to come back later, to postpone your decision.

19. Eventually you come back out into the sunlight and step across the stream once more. The world seems very beautiful in the soft late afternoon sun. You feel the earth beneath your feet and give thanks for the gifts of life. You remember the people you love and give thanks for good relationships. You ponder what is good and fine in your life and determine you won't take it for granted again. You ponder what is bad and think how you will manage to transform it. Now you have been on the meat-hook, there are no trials you cannot face. You have been to the underworld, met your shadow and given up the delusions of life. Now you can be re-born...

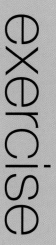

exercise

CHAPTER THIRTEEN

DEATH

Death. The final taboo. We live our lives trying to ignore it, to push it away, to pretend it won't happen – at least not to us. Yet the unpalatable and inescapable truth is that we all die – every single one of us. Our attempts to shy away from death would be comic if they weren't so tragic. I remember interviewing a bunch of people who firmly believed that they were immortal, that they alone would never die. They were delightful people, full of vigour and verve – they were also in the prime of life. A few years later I bumped into one of them by accident and inquired after one of his co-immortalists. 'Ah,' said the man, 'um, er, he died. Car accident.' It was sad but it was also blackly humorous – of course he died. He shouldn't have died so soon but it was a delusion to imagine he could dodge death. A delusion based on fear. So why are we so frightened of death?

People who have had near-death experiences talk in terms energyworkers can understand. They see lights, hear sounds, feel themselves uplifted, filled with transcendent energy, pulled towards a source of power and light and energy.

I think our fears come about because we think of ourselves in terms of our egos, our personality. Most of us spend our lives bolstering our egos, surrounding ourselves with symbols of security and status – we build a comfort cocoon to block away anything unpleasant or unsavoury. We keep ourselves busy, frenetically busy (whether that involves working like crazy or vegging out in front of a television) – we will do almost anything to avoid thinking about life and, more importantly death and what awaits us there. We are scared of losing our friends, our families, our pets, our homes, our standing in life. The fear comes about because we have not grasped the most important fact about energy. We are not ego-bound individuals, but part of the universal whole. People who have had near-death experiences talk in terms energyworkers can understand. They see lights, hear sounds, feel themselves uplifted, filled with transcendent energy, pulled towards a source of power and light and energy. Ancient traditions such as the Egyptian, Indian and Tibetan all talk of the various energy bodies that are released in death, allowing the soul finally to escape its material shackles and become pure energy once more. When we die we ascend the Tree of Life, becoming purer and purer energy as we leave behind our material shell.

As energy beings we are not separate from life or death – we are not ego-bound individuals struggling on our own;

we are part of the whole, the universal energy source

DEATHWORKING

The paradoxical point about death is that it can make life so much better. If you decide not to shy away from death but spend time working with death energy, you can invest your life with all the energy that would otherwise have been wasted in locking away your fear. Again and again you hear about people who find out they only have a matter of months, or even weeks, to live. Instead of rolling over and sinking into depression, they decide they will make the most of this last time. Many discover wonderful truths about themselves: they uncover huge reserves of strength, power, character. Some find amazing routes to healing and don't even die then at all. But all say that the thought of dying focuses the spirit like nothing else. Of course you don't have to wait until the doctor gives you the bad news – you could start right now...

exercise

A YEAR TO LIVE

This exercise is incredibly powerful. If you have followed the Inanna descent from the previous chapter, you should find you have already done the groundwork. But even if you find it distasteful, do try to put aside some time to consider the following.

● Imagine you only had one year left to live. How would you spend that year? What would you do? What would be most important? What would not be important?

● Would you give up your work or change your job?

● Who would you see more of; who would you see less of?

● Write letters to all those people you love and cherish. Tell them how important they have been to you. Tell them what you appreciate about them. Maybe you should send these letters – now, before it's too late.

● Consider those people you don't get on with. Are there any people you hold grudges against, anyone you have an ongoing feud with? Do you want to take this negative energy with you when you die? If not, now's the time to put things to right. Again, a letter might be best – write down your feelings. Be honest but fair. Try to understand their point of view. Can you clear this karmic debt?

● Who could you help in this last year? Who could benefit from your time, your energy, your money? Why not try to help them now?

● Review your life. Is there anything you regret not doing? Anything you always wanted to do? Why not think about doing it now?

● Did you make any mistakes? Could you put them right? If not, let them go, don't waste energy on them. If there's something that could be done, why put it off?

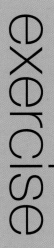

You see, death focuses the mind like almost nothing else. What would you do if you had only a month to live? A week to live? A day to live? An hour to live? Why not live every day as if it were your last? Use death energy to create life – live consciously, enjoy every moment, don't have regrets. Try not to put things off indefinitely. I'm not suggesting we all go out on a giant shopping spree, or pack up work or ditch a relationship. But I am suggesting you think about what is really important. Don't imagine you have limitless time. If your work doesn't work for you, look at the suggestions in Part Three, Chapter Three. If your relationships aren't serving you well, spend some time with Part Two. Maybe it is time to move on, but equally it may just be time for more honestly, more communication. Do it now, don't let it fester. Before you know it you might be old and bitter, regretting a lifetime of wasted opportunities.

exercise

FACING FEAR

We all have pretty much the same fears. The only difference is how we face them.
If we shy away from them, they grab the opportunity to grow, huge and faceless in our subconscious. If we face them bravely and squarely, they can be a stepping stone to huge growth. Spend five minutes a day solidly facing your fears.

Start with your small everyday fears. Observe your fears, watch them – figure out that many of them are unnecessary or mere indulgences.

● Now move onto the big fears. What is your greatest fear? What is the worst thing that you could imagine happening to you?

● Why would it be so awful? See if you can reduce your fears down to manageable proportions. Most come down to fear of lack of security (losing possessions, home, job); lack of love (losing dear ones, not having relationships), lack of face (making a fool of yourself, appearing stupid).

● The key is to remember the ebb and flow of energy. We are energetic beings living in an energetic world. When people die they do not really leave us; they are just no longer in their physical, gross, material bodies. We cannot reach out and hug them bodily but they can still touch our hearts. If you lost everything, would it be so awful? The universe might have some new lesson for you. Many people who lose everything find that, in retrospect, it can be a huge push towards growth. Generally there IS a reason for everything in life.

My favorite quote regarding death comes from Stephen Levine, author of *Who Dies?* and *A Year to Live* (both highly recommended). Levine worked with terminally ill patients for over 20 years. He says, 'Of course, the reason that some part of us denies that it will die is because it never does...the reason something within feels immortal is because it is.' From an Eastern viewpoint the concept of death simply doesn't exist. We just move from one state of being to another; from one kind of energy to a different kind. As we have seen throughout this book, the universe is pure consciousness, pure energy – once you die you simply remove many of the veils that prevent us from seeing the true nature of being.

A sad piece of synchronicity happened as I was writing this. At just this point I had to stop writing to take my cat, Bear (she who loves the dancing rainbows), to the vet. Over the last week she had suddenly become unwell, refusing to eat and becoming very listless. As I watched her I knew she was dying. The vet confirmed that she had total renal failure and that the only kind thing to do was to put her to sleep. We agreed and I held her, stroking her and talking to her as he administered the injection. What stunned me was that I knew the very second she died. One moment she was Bear, inhabiting her body; the next 'Bear' just wasn't there any more. The body had become a shell. Her vital energy, her spirit, had departed. Now, as I write this, there is a little cat-sized gap in my life. I keep expecting to hear her insistent miaow, to feel her jump up on the bed, to come racing out to greet us as we arrive home. It made me remember my first cat, Pip, who lived to the ripe old age of 18. He died when I was about seven and my mother tried to accustom me to not having him around by saying he was ill and staying at the vet. That night I heard a scratching at my bedroom window. I opened the window and there was Pip. I stroked him and cuddled him but he wouldn't come in the house so I went to sleep with the window open. Years later my mother told me she remembered asking me why I had the window wide open in the middle of winter. When I told her about Pip she couldn't believe it. He couldn't have come to visit me because he was dead.

Even had it been another cat, she reasoned, how did it climb a sheer wall to a first-floor window? Surely to comfort and reassure the child he loved? Rest assured there is an energy that survives death.

WHERE WERE YOU BEFORE YOU WERE BORN?

If the idea of death still frightens you, think about this question. Who were you before you were born? Where were you? Look into a small baby's eyes and there is usually something strange and knowing in them – if only they could tell us what they have seen, where they have come from. We've all been through birth: we survived! We came from somewhere into this body, this life – and we will depart from this body, this life back to that place. The mystery is that we cannot remember – although some people reckon they have been given an insight. Rebirthing, which we discussed in Part Two, takes you, through a specific breathing exercise, back to the original birth process. Many people find they can go back further still, to the point of conception. I wouldn't recommend anyone use the rebirthing breathing on their own – you should see a qualified therapist. But you might find you can achieve similar results with this exercise.

exercise

1. Find a place where you won't be disturbed and where you can be comfortable and warm. Lie down and relax your body, checking each part – from the top of your head to your toes (not forgetting the shoulders, jaw, hands and all those places you know you collect tension!) – is relaxed.

2. Focus on your breath, just watching it for a few minutes. Notice how gradually it becomes slower and calmer, slower and deeper. Start breathing into your solar plexus and notice how that feels. As you breathe in, know you are taking in new life and energy. As you breathe out, allow yourself to let go of all your fear – imagine your fears dispersing like leaves in the wind.

3. When you feel quite relaxed and are breathing slowly and deeply, start to go back through your life. Review where you are now – what you are doing, who you are with, how you feel. Then slowly scroll back through your adult life – don't dwell or judge; just review.

4. Take yourself back to your teenage years. Then to your childhood. What do you remember? What was important? Can you recall your first day at school? Where was your first home? How far back can you remember?

5. When you reach as far back as you can, start to imagine. Imagine yourself as a toddler, as a baby. If you have seen photographs, put yourself into them. Pretend you remember.

6. You are lying in your pram. Now go back further still. You are being born. You are being pushed down through the birth canal, squeezed and pressed into life. You emerge into the world and open your mouth to breathe – and scream! Stay with this for a while – how does it feel?

7. Now go back further. You are in the womb, warm, enclosed, surrounded by the gentle waters of the amniotic fluid. You hear your mother's heartbeat above you, the gurgling of her stomach, the sway of her walk. As you float you can remember all manner of things – you can easily go back still further to a time when you were not even in physical form.

8. You are in the other place. How does it feel? How do you feel? Spend some time just being in this pure energy form. Feel the freedom.

9. Now remember why you decided to come back to earth, to a physical form. From a distance you see your parents-to-be. What made you choose them? What lessons did you all need to learn? Your parentage was no accident – it was a conscious decision. So why did you make it? Stay with this thought for some time – it may give you some very valuable insights.

10. When you feel you have learned all you can, slowly bring your awareness back to your breath. Become aware of the room around you – your body lying on the floor. Hear the sounds around you. Gently open your eyes. Lie still for a few moments then slowly get up and stamp your feet. You may want to have a warm drink and a biscuit to ground you completely. Record your experiences in your journal.

exercise

Realizing that you decided to be born, that you decided on your parents and your situation in life, can be very liberating. Once again we have to realize that we are in control of our own lives, our own destinies. We have to take responsibility. Seemingly terrible things may have happened to us but at some level we decided to go through these experiences. We wanted to learn. What lessons are you here to learn? Will you ensure they are learned before you die or will you miss the opportunity?

THE DARK PATH

Many spiritual teachings advise that we 'practise' dying, that we walk many times the path we will take when we die. So that the soul, when confronted with death, is not unprepared but automatically follows the process. There are various techniques and rituals but I like, once again, to use a qabalistic pathworking. This path takes the temple of Malkuth as its starting point and descends to the realm of Hades, Lord of the Underworld. Although it sounds dark and gloomy it is in fact, once again, a wonderful chance for growth and self-knowledge. It is a form of initiation into the mysteries of Life and Death – we need to be able to plumb our own depths to be able to enjoy our own heights. We need to understand that we are all part of a natural rhythm, that our energy pulses to a universal pattern. This pathworking is a natural progression from the Inanna descent we made in the last chapter. It teaches us that in order to discover new life we have to discard the old. We have to search for the light in the darkest of places.

There is also another purpose for this ritual. I like to take this journey when anyone I know dies. By doing so, you can take the opportunity to talk with them, to finish any 'unfinished business'. You can also help them make the transition to their new life – if they become stuck, as some people do, in fear and trepidation. It is also a great service to perform this ritual if there has been a disaster in which a lot of people died suddenly and unexpectedly. Many such souls feel lost and become 'stuck' in the shadows. You can help them move across.
Are you ready? Let's take another visit to the underworld...

exercise

1. We start in the Temple of Malkuth. Spend some time building the temple as we did on page 170 Greet Sandalphon and approach the altar. On it you notice there is a wide bronze bowl which contains a pile of silver coins. Take a handful and put them in the deep pocket of your robe.

2. Between the pillars you see the tarot card of The World. As you watch the curtain it becomes three-dimensional; the colours swirl and you walk forwards into it and through it. As we walk through we find ourselves in the same landscape as in the previous chapter, for our descent with Inanna. You walk across fields of swaying corn, dotted with poppies and cornflowers. Birds are singing and the sun shines brightly. The whole world seems beautiful and once

again part of you yearns to sit and enjoy the bounty of the natural world, then to return home. But you see ahead of you the familiar range of mountains, and you know that, once again, your quest leads you there.

3. You come to a fast-flowing stream over which lie stepping stones, leading to a dark cave. As you walk into the shadow of the rocks, you feel a chill run over your body but you continue bravely. You step into the cave and it seems as though all the light and warmth of the world has vanished.

4. At the back of the cave is one small lamp. A voice speaks out from the gloom; it is Hecate, the crone, the wise woman. She asks you why you have come and you tell her that you wish to descend to the kingdom of Persephone and Hades. She points to a small opening at the back of the cave and gives you the lamp to guide your way.

5. You squeeze through the opening and find yourself in a small tunnel which runs steeply downwards. The walls close in around you and you feel quite claustrophobic. As you follow the path, you can feel the living rock around you, pressing in against you, almost squeezing you, as if you were being born. The path is difficult: sometimes you have to crawl along, sometimes squeeze through narrow stretches. But finally the path opens out and you find yourself in a vast cavern, lit by flickering torches.

6. The ground beneath your feet is fine sand and you realize you are standing on the shore of a great river. On the edge of the river is a boat and by it stands Charon, the ferryman of the dead. Around him throng the souls of the dead, those who cannot make the crossing. You pause and see if there is anyone here you know. If so, you can talk to them and resolve any unfinished business. When you feel content, say your farewells and give them one of your silver coins so they can cross the river.

7. If there isn't anyone you know you should pass out your coins to the others. Bless them and send them on their way back to the source of all energy. Keep back two coins for yourself. Hand one to Charon and get in his boat. Slowly he rows across the river and you get out on the other side.

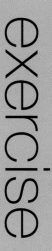

exercise

8. Before you stand gates which swing open as you approach. In a great hall there are two thrones on which sit Hades and Persephone, Lord and Lady of the Underworld. You walk forwards until you stand before the couple and look into their eyes. Surprisingly they are not stern or terrifying but kind and laughing. You realize they are not just the King and Queen of the Dead but the Lord and Lady of Rebirth. They welcome you with pleasure.

9. Hades leads you to a mirror and asks you to look into it. Within it you see your true self, as it was before you took bodily form and as it will be after you relinquish your body. What do you see? What is your true essence? You realize that beyond our looks, our personality, our hopes and fears, our possessions, lies the real us – a timeless, deathless, energetic essence.

10. Persephone steps forward and embraces you warmly. You feel your real essence shine through as your body seems to disappear and you and she feel as if you were floating up and up, towards the stars. Then you seem to become the stars themselves. You shimmer with energy, with joy, with love and a pure sense of bliss.

11. Gently she breathes on your face and tells you that it is not yet time to become a being of pure energy, to rejoin the source of all Love and Light. Softly she carries you down again to the great hall and bids you farewell for now.

12. Smiling, you take your leave and retrace your steps. Charon accepts your other silver coin and takes you back across the lake. You promise the souls waiting that you will return with more coins. You find your way back to the cave swiftly and easily. Hecate takes the lamp and smiles. You look into her eyes and can no longer tell if she is an old woman or a young girl.

13. As you walk out of the cave your eyes blink to adjust to the sudden light. All around you the world seems very beautiful and you resolve to enjoy your life, and make the most of what is left of it. Before you stand two trees and between them is the tarot card curtain of The World, as before. You step through it and back to the Temple of Malkuth.

14. Sandalphon greets you and you spend a few moments sharing your experience with him and giving thanks. He reminds you that you should walk this path often – for yourself but also for the lost souls who have forgotten their connection to the Source.

CLAIMING OUR ENERGETIC HERITAGE

The more we investigate our own dark energy, the more we face our fears and confront our own deaths, the more we will find we live. Most of us curtail our energy with our fears and suspicions: we half-live. Releasing the fear of death and discovering our true nature is a huge liberation.

The Energy Secret isn't really a 'secret' at all – it is something that is out there for all of us to share. In the years to come I am quite sure that working with energy will seem the most natural thing in all the world.

The path we have followed in this book has been a curious one. I hope you have found it as beneficial and eye-opening as I have. By now you have probably realized that The Energy Secret isn't really a 'secret' at all – it is something that is out there for all of us to share. In the years to come I am quite sure that working with energy will seem the most natural thing in all the world. In fact it will seem strange not to use this wonderful power, this essence, to its full capacity. For without a knowledge of, and use of, our own energy, we just don't live to our full potential. Incorporating energy into your everyday life makes each day an adventure, a learning process, a further step on our lifelong path. It starts simply, by helping us get in touch with our bodies and discover better health. It progresses by informing our relationships – with ourselves, with each other, with friends, family, work colleagues, even complete strangers. It ends by linking us with our spirituality, our eternal nature as beings of pure energy and light. It is a path of great joy but also sadness. Sometimes it is easy, sometimes difficult and painful. But as we begin to feel energy moving in our bodies and in our lives, we start to discover the true secret. We begin to know ourselves for what we truly are – we understand the nature of our being and our true heritage. We learn to live with energy, to work with energy, to be energy.

I hope you enjoy the journey and look forward to meeting you – as we all will meet – at the source of all energy and light.

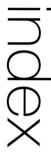

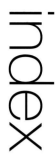

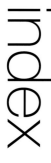

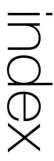

bibliography

HEALING

The Five Minute Healer
by Jane Alexander (Gaia)
The Detox Plan
by Jane Alexander (Gaia)
Healing Mind, Healthy Woman
by Alice D Domar and Henry Dreher
(Thorsons)
Your Body Speaks your Mind
by Debbie Shapiro (Piatkus)
Vibrational Medicine by Richard Gerber
(Bear & Co)
Living in Balance by Joel Levey and
Michelle Levey (Conari)
Simple Meditation and Relaxation
by Joel Levey and Michelle Levey
(Conari)
The Complete Healer by David Furlong
(Piatkus)
Healers and Healing by Roy Stemman
(Piatkus)
The God Experiment
by Russell Stannard (Faber)
Healing with Sound
by Olivea Dewhurst-Maddock (Gaia)
Healing with Colour
by Theo Gimbel (Gaia)
Shiatsu by Elaine Liechti (Element)

CHAKRAS

Eastern Body, Western Mind
by Anodea Judith (Celestial Arts)
Opening to Spirit
by Caroline Shola Arewa (Thorsons)
The Rainbow Journey
by Dr Brenda Davies
(Hodder & Stoughton)

FLOWER REMEDIES

The Twelve Healers & Other Remedies
by Edward Bach (C W Daniel)
Heal Thyself by Edward Bach
(C W Daniel)
Bach Flower Remedies for Women
by Judy Howard (C W Daniel)

FOOD

The Ancient Cookfire
by Carrie L'Esperance (Bear & Co)
Feeding the Body, Nourishing the Soul
by Deborah Kesten (Conari)

Healing Drinks by Anne McIntyre (Gaia)

EXERCISE

A Woman's Guide to Tantra Yoga
by Vimala McClure
(New World Library)
Body, Mind and Sport by John Douillard
(Harmony Books)
Chi Kung for Health and Vitality
by Wong Kiew Kit (Element)
Yoga for Stress Relief
by Swami Shivapremananda (Gaia)
The Big Book of Ch'I by Paul Wildish
(Thorsons)

EMOTIONAL ENERGY

Sacred Fire by Tiziana de Rovere
(Celestial Arts)
The Dance of Intimacy
by Harriet Lerner (Thorsons)

PSYCHIC PROTECTION

Spiritual Cleansing by Draja Mickaharic
(Weiser)
The Art of Psychic Protection
by Judy Hall (Findhorn Press)

SEXUAL ENERGY

Tantric Yoga by Gavin and Yvonne Frost
(Weiser)
The Art of Sexual Magic
by Margo Anand (Piatkus)
*Barefoot Doctor's Handbook for Modern
Lovers* (Piatkus)

ENERGY IN THE HOME

Spirit of the Home by Jane Alexander
(Thorsons)
The Illustrated Spirit of the Home
by Jane Alexander (Thorsons)
A Home for the Soul by Anthony Lawlor
(Potter)

NATURAL ENERGY

The Natural Year by Jane Alexander
(Avon)
The Spirit of Place by Loren Cruden
(Destiny Books)
The Healing Energies of Water
by Charlie Ryrie (Gaia)

CITY AND WORKPLACE ENERGY

The Work we were Born to Do
by Nick Williams (Element)
Feng Shui at Work
by Kirsten M Lagatree (Newleaf)
Creating the Work You Love
by Rick Jarow (Destiny Books)
The Seed Handbook by Lynne Franks
(Thorsons)
The Urban Warrior's Book of Solutions
by Dr Michael McGannon (Arrow)

SPIRITUAL ENERGY

The Smudge Pack by Jane Alexander
(Thorsons)
Rituals for Sacred Living
by Jane Alexander (Thorsons)
The Stormy Search for the Self
by Christina and Stanislav Grof
(Thorsons)

QABALAH

Opening the Inner Gates edited by
Edward Hoffman (Shambhala)
The Living Qabalah by Will Parfitt
(Element)
The Essential Kabbalah
by Daniel C Matt (HarperCollins)

DARK ENERGY

Romancing the Shadow
by Connie Zweig and Steve Wolf
(Thorsons)
Owning Your Own Shadow
by Robert A Johnson
(Harper SanFrancisco)
*The Middle Passage – from Misery to
Meaning in Midlife* by James Hollis
(Inner City Books)

DEATH ENERGY

Deathing by Anya Foos-Graber
(Nicholas Hays)
Death: Beginning or End
by Dr Jonn Mumford (Llewellyn)
Facing Death and Finding Hope
by Christine Longaker (Arrow)